The Expert's Guide to Nutrition
on a Plant-based Diet

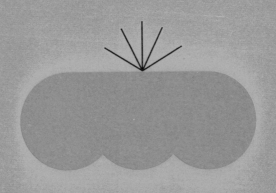

Vegan
Savvy

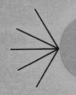

Azmina Govindji RD

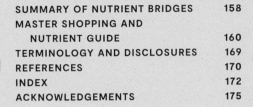

Seven

Boost Your Energy

P.74

Savvy tips to feel
more energised by
improving iron absorption,
eating foods rich in B-vitamins
and giving your body
enough fuel.

Ten

Eating In: Building Healthy Habits at Home

P.136

What to look for when shopping, how
to compare brands and get the scoop
on convenience foods, plus my top
plant-for-animal swaps and how to
make decisions when planning meals.

Eight

Calcium Without Dairy

P.94

Why vegan alternatives
to dairy aren't always
a good nutritional substitute,
especially when it comes
to calcium, plus how to
meet your daily calcium
requirements with simple
swaps and additions.

Eleven

Eating Out: Staying Powerful When Out and About

P.146

Tips and tricks to help you make your
favourite meals healthier whether you're
grabbing lunch on the go or dining
out in style.

Nine

Micronutrients: Small but Mighty

P.114

Simple ways to sprinkle on your B12, crunch
through your iodine and stir in your zinc.

Twelve

Beyond the Book: Bringing It All Together

P.154

Need a master shopping and nutrition
guide? Sorted. Instant guide to which
foods have what nutrients?
Done. All your Nutrient
Bridges in one place?
You've got it.

'While spelling it all out, Gil sometimes literally spells it out. He likes to emphasise a point by spelling the key word. He likes to break words down for me, crack them open, reveal the knowledge inside, like the meat inside a nut. *Calorie*, for instance. He says it comes from the Latin *calor*, which is a measure of heat. People think calories are bad, Gil says, but calories are just measures of heat, and we need heat. With food, you feed your body's natural furnace. How can that be bad? It's *when* you eat, *how much* you eat, the *choices* you make – that's what makes all the difference. People think eating is bad, he says, but we need to stoke our internal fire.'

— Andre Agassi, OPEN, An Autobiography

Introduction

This book is about enjoying food, *not* restricting it. There's no need to cut carbs, fear fats or count calories. Veganism is about more than just food and my aim is to enrich the dietary part of your lifestyle. There are various definitions of a plant-based diet, ranging from one devoid of any animal products (vegan), to one that is predominantly, but not exclusively, based on plant foods. This book is about 100% plant-based eating but the tips and tricks for getting nutritional balance will be helpful to the whole family, whether you're vegan or not.

It's easy to be an unhealthy vegan. You could have sugar-rich drinks and fast foods every day and still follow a plant-based diet. It's not only the famous vitamin B12 that deserves attention – there are other micronutrients, such as iodine and omega-3 fatty acids, that need to be considered in a vegan eating plan.

The jolt that spurred me into action

I've spent my life researching hot diet topics, combatting fake news and guiding people towards making better, sustainable dietary choices. As a media spokesperson for the British Dietetic Association and TV nutritionist, I've constantly strived to be on top of the latest trends and research. But then something changed. I vividly remember standing in the kitchen four years ago when my 23 year-old daughter Shazia announced she had become vegan – and all of a sudden it got personal. Her decision really concerned me, especially because young girls already tend not to have enough calcium and iodine, and now she could be even more compromised. The drive and energy I put into learning about vegan diets came from a different place as I now had a vested interest. The idea of writing down my nutrition hacks for Shazia and vegans like her was born.

Having started this project primarily in my role as a mother to help keep my daughter healthy, the professional dietitian in me became increasingly inspired to find creative ways to make daily eating more nutritious for all vegans. I wanted to keep writing to create an evidence-based resource for all vegans to help them to embrace the goodness and deliciousness of whole plant foods. After all, you can get all essential nutrients from well-planned vegan diets!

My eight-week plant-based trial

I am not vegan. But I always test out diets before writing a book, so I trialled 100% plant-based eating while doing my research. Like any new way of eating, it took a fair bit of adjustment. I realised quite quickly that failing to plan ahead was not a good idea. It would have been easy to opt for nothing but salads or soup, but that wasn't going to fill me up, would have been pretty boring, and would be lacking in essential nutrients.

So, I planned. I created a shopping list, I wrote down meal ideas that we enjoyed as a family – stir-fries, curries, pasta, roasted vegetables, quick meals made from convenient shortcuts, and so on. Once I'd got the basics right, I needed to satisfy my nutritional curiosity by checking how well-balanced the meals were. I found that I was in danger of being low in nutrients I normally wouldn't even think about, such as iron from red meat, omega-3 fats from oily fish, and iodine from dairy products. I gave up drinking tea with meals (tannins in tea inhibit the absorption of iron from vegetables), I added nuts and seeds to dishes to top up my protein, and I found I needed a lot more time in the supermarket to scrutinise food labels. To my dismay, I observed that many plant-based drinks don't have added iodine or vitamin B12, many vegan cheeses don't have added calcium and give you little protein, and countless vegan ready meals are nutritionally unbalanced. Vegan choices are often more expensive too.

I thought about how to fill the nutrient gaps with fortified foods. I made umami-tasting soups using savoury yeast extract spread or miso for B vitamins and zinc, and mixed bean chilli flavoured with nutritional yeast flakes for my vitamin B12. I conjured up quick and easy recipes that offered me enough protein, vitamins and minerals, and I drank a little orange juice with meals to enhance my iron absorption. I started to feel energised – I wasn't hungry, and my meals became colourful and exciting.

I've scouted the shops, read labels, researched the latest studies, analysed vegan foods and created shopping lists in order to show you how to fill potential nutrient gaps. This book is a combination of insights from both the mother and the diligent healthcare professional in me. I've finally found a way to give Shazia realistic advice that comes from a deeper place within me. I continue to grow and learn, and that learning is what I have put into these pages. I hope you like it, and good luck!

Azmina x

How to read this book

Being vegan savvy is about eating delicious meals while being aware of the different factors that affect how your body can make the best use of nutrients from plant-based foods. You can read this book cover-to-cover and take a comprehensive tour of the best and simplest ways to move towards an energised and balanced way of plant-based eating. However, you might be more of a dip-in, dip-out kind of reader and that's fine too. Besides the first two chapters, each chapter is complete in itself, so you won't feel lost if you read them in a different order. Whichever way you read this book, there are two important bedrocks that you should start with:

1. *Getting Your Mind on Your Side* gives you simple, tried and tested behavioural psychology tips to help you achieve the results you want.
2. *Picture Your Plate* will equip you with the foundational principles of nutrition that the rest of the book builds upon.

The nutrient bridge

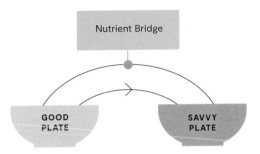

This Nutrient Bridge is a unique tool devised for this book to help you make simple changes that will enrich your meals.

When you become vegan, it's natural to start experimenting with plant-based alternatives: you might try dairy-free cheese and milk substitutes or vegan ready-meals. But it's important to understand that cutting out meat and dairy doesn't automatically mean you'll be healthier. On the contrary, you could be missing out on essential vitamins and minerals that your body needs on a daily basis, like calcium, iron, omega-3 fats and iodine, as well as the more obvious vitamin B12. So, there could be a 'gap' in the nutrients you are getting – I call this the 'nutrient gap'.

In this book, you'll find Nutrient Bridges – simple tips to help you get the nutrients you might otherwise be lacking, thereby bridging the nutrient gap. They're easy tricks, like stir-frying carrots instead of eating them raw to help your body convert beta-carotene into vitamin A. Some bridges are swaps, like cooking with rapeseed oil instead of coconut oil to reduce your saturated fat intake, while others are small additions to your meals, like adding a handful of nuts for omega-3 fats or a few sheets of roasted seaweed for iodine. Some Nutrient Bridges double up as ways to add flavour – a sprinkling of nutritional yeast, for example, is not only a great source of vitamin B12 but also adds a delicious umami taste.

The iron nutrient bridge: an example

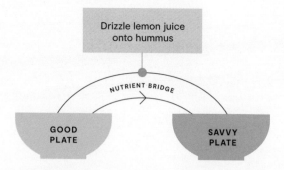

If you're eating hummus with pitta bread, drizzling on lemon juice will help your body to make use of the iron in the chickpeas. This is a simple way to visualise that. The aim is to take you from a 'good plate' to a 'savvy plate'. All the Nutrient Bridges are also listed in the last chapter for handy access.

'Nutrition should never be a problem if you're well informed and motivated.'

Rely on the research

Each chapter is underpinned and substantiated by considerable research, with references listed at the back of the book. Many of the research summaries are based on robust studies and form part of national dietary guidelines. Others are smaller studies as there haven't been many strong studies on vegans and the number of people in the studies are still relatively small. They do, however, highlight where the evidence is pointing and there's no doubt that over time researchers will build on this knowledge, especially as plant-based eating gains momentum. I keep a close watch on new developments in vegan diets and share my views on my website and social media channels.

RESEARCH

In each chapter you'll see research summaries in boxes like these.

Dotted throughout the book you'll find *Thought Lifters*. It may not always be easy to digest and put into practice some of the nutritional insights, so I've included these to help you along your way.

However you read this book, remember to trust your instincts and follow what stands out for you. Take small steps towards incorporating the advice that feels achievable and build on this over time as you embrace your new healthier lifestyle. I'd love to hear how you're getting on: write to me via azminanutrition.com or on @AzminaNutrition on Twitter or Instagram. Thank you for choosing *Vegan Savvy*, enjoy!

THOUGHT LIFTER

Choose to be grateful for all the times you've eaten well rather than guilty for the times you didn't manage it. Focus your attention on your successes.

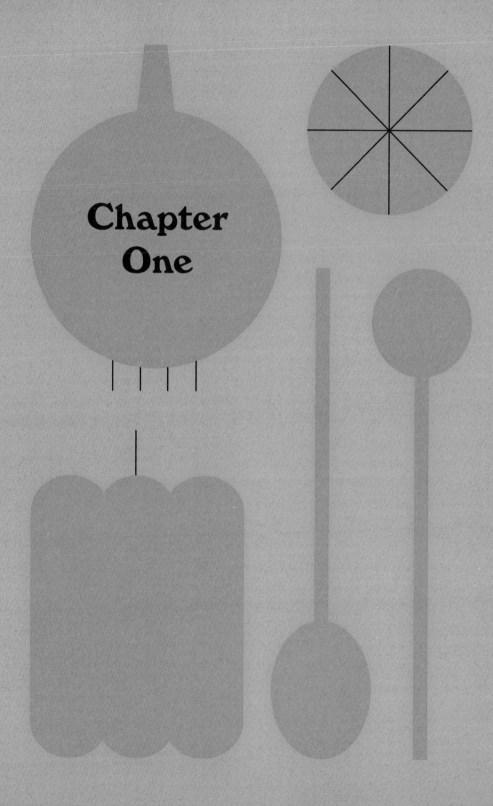

Chapter
One

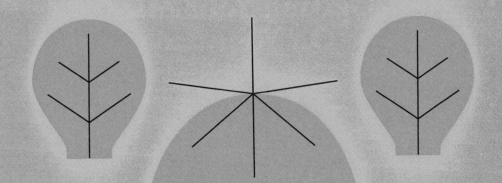

Getting Your Mind on Your Side

Getting Your Mind On Your Side

Whenever you set out to make changes in your eating habits, make sure your mind is on board too. Even with the best advice, you're likely to get limited results unless you've prepared yourself mentally with a positive and resourceful mindset. If you're serious about making a fundamental shift in the way you eat, this needs to be realistic in order for it to last.

Harnessing the power of your mind can lead to sustainable changes, so take a few short minutes now to really internalise the value that this lifestyle change will bring. You may want to have more energy for the gym, enjoy more variety when you're eating out, or perhaps something more life-enhancing like improving your relationships or long-term health. You might find that doing this improves your confidence and likelihood of success, especially if you write down what comes to mind and re-read it often.

Having dipped into the behavioural research from Nudge Theory[1], I've learned that we tend to subconsciously follow what others are doing; whether that's our peers or people we don't know. Concepts like Veganuary may be conducive to this sort of herd behaviour: people might go vegan for a month because others are doing so. It can also be more motivating to know you're not in it alone.

Build on this concept to explore your own behaviours and motivations, for example by finding people who are also starting a vegan diet, or who have been vegan for years and want to eat better. You could share recipes, seek out healthier vegan products together, and celebrate each other's successes.

There is some research on how the position of foods visually on a plate may affect eating experience. It has been suggested that when food is arranged more neatly on a plate, this influences how much people like the meal[2]. We know that monitoring the portion size of unhealthy foods is conducive to better eating. The VVPC plate (chapter 2), on which this book is based, is a clever way of increasing the portion size of nutritious vegetables and salads, while adding colour and visual appeal to your meal. If you decide to position your meal components in the vegetable, protein

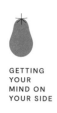

or carbs location of your plate, you might find this adds a different dimension to your eating experience, bringing with it a neater plate and perhaps more mindfulness.

We don't just eat when we're hungry

Feeling sad, angry or guilty may make you less inclined to eat better. You may reach for a biscuit or a pack of crisps for comfort. This behaviour might be an indication that you're at a vulnerable point, making you more likely to make poor eating choices. Uncompromising willpower isn't available to any of us *all* of the time, so the first step is just to notice when you are eating in response to your emotions.

SAVVY TIP

The next time you find yourself craving unhealthy foods, do something to help break your current state of mind. One of the best ways to do that is to physically move away from where you are. Stand up and walk around the room, put on an upbeat tune and dance for 20 seconds, or lie on the floor and do some stretching. You could also try deep breathing, phoning a friend, or distracting yourself with a task. Simply moving from a seated position to standing tall might be all it takes to help you resist temptation and let a craving pass. The visualisation technique on page 15 might also help.

The *Thought Lifters* dotted throughout are intended to give you a mental boost, a momentary distraction from any negativity. Having a more positive state of mind may pave the way for making healthier eating more pleasurable. In time, you will start to feel more energised and being vegan savvy will become an integral part of how you eat.

Conscious shopping

Research suggests that the food choices we make are influenced by how available and accessible that food is, and also whether it's affordable[3]. Most of the foods I recommend are basic everyday foods such as wholegrains, fruits, vegetables, beans and lentils. You'll also see tips on getting nutrient boosts, for example, by choosing rapeseed oil in cooking for omega-3 fatty acids, or fortified breakfast cereals as a source of iron.

Other foods I recommend may appear less regularly on your shopping list, and may also be less accessible, affordable and available.

Examples are B12 nutritional yeast flakes, iodine-providing roasted seaweed and selenium-rich Brazil nuts. However, I encourage you to go the extra mile with these as you only need small amounts to make up nutrition gaps in a vegan diet. Make these foods regular items on your shopping list, so they become accessible whenever you're cooking or need a snack. Some may only be available online, but as plant-based eating becomes more mainstream, I would expect that you'll soon see these on the supermarket shelves.

SAVVY TIP

Keep healthful foods within easy reach in your kitchen.

Write it down

As you're reading this book, if something triggers an '*aha*' moment, make a note of it. Do this often and keep this list handy so you can remind yourself of ideas or thoughts that work for you. In particular, jotting down your successes helps to keep them front of mind to give you a lift.

What inspires me about becoming a savvy vegan?

Consider what mindset you want to be in when you start this journey. Here are five simple questions to ask yourself – some people find that writing down the answers helps them to focus.

1. How will improving the way I eat benefit me?
2. What is truly important to me about making this change?
3. How much happier will I feel once I'm confident that I'm on the right track?
4. How would this new lifestyle benefit other areas of my life?
5. What impact might this have on significant people around me?

THOUGHT LIFTER

Just do your best to take on these tips and accept that sometimes it may not all go to plan. That's life! The learning is in the stumbling.

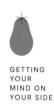

Some people find that imagining themselves as the person they aspire to be can be a strong motivator. If this is you, here's a quick visualisation technique:

1. Close your eyes and imagine yourself as your 'new' you. Energised, happy and healthy.
2. What are you wearing? What else do you see in the picture?
3. Are there any sounds? Conversations, birds, and so on?
4. Make your image even brighter by adding rich colours and more pleasing sounds.
5. What are you feeling? Stay there for a while... enjoy it.

You can use this image to inspire you to make the changes you desire. A drawing of something that represents the new you might help bring it to life. This can be as simple as a graceful bird or a tall palm tree. Or an inspiring song, a poster; anything that can be a metaphor for the new you. Hang it on the fridge door or by your desk at work. You have control over your thoughts and actions.

Having said that, don't be too hard on yourself. Dietary change isn't something that people try out for a few days and find they're able to sustain forever without effort. Just like working out at the gym needs repetition, conditioning and practice, so does dietary change. Be kind to yourself, take baby steps. And if at times you feel like giving up on your goals, bring up your metaphor or visualisation to give you a spark of motivation and remind yourself why you started.

You might want to start by setting yourself a tiny goal. It could be to drink one glass of water a day, to eat one piece of fruit, to chew your first mouthful of a meal slowly and consciously. The key is to start small and build a habit rather than get everything right at the outset.

Further, becoming accountable to someone other than yourself might increase your chances of success. It can be easy to get in a slump and let yourself down, but you may have a different level of commitment if you're at risk of letting someone else down. Is there a friend or family member who could support and encourage you?

THOUGHT LIFTER

Simple nudges from a trusted friend once a week or once a day can help you stick to new habits.

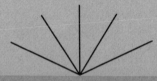

Chapter
Two

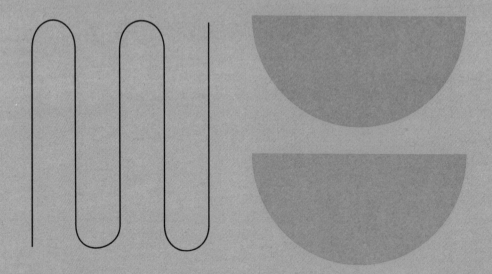

Picture Your Plate

Picture your plate

Many people get bogged down by all the health information out there: from government recommendations and food labels, to features in magazines and ever-changing 'superfood' claims. They find it so complex that it starts to feel impossible to know what to eat to be healthy, and it can be particularly confusing for people with other health conditions like diabetes, heart disease, raised blood cholesterol or obesity.

So I came up with a simple, visual and memorable solution to empower people to know what to eat and feel confident that they're making the right choices at mealtimes. I scouted various studies, publications and respected nutrition guides to ensure my ideas had substance and were based on evidence, and landed on a model that is effective yet simple enough for everyone to grasp. I have been using it for over fifteen years with my patients, as well as in my previous books, and am humbled by the overwhelmingly positive feedback. I consistently hear from people that the mental image has stuck with them and helped to simplify the way they think about meals. It has even given many a sense of confidence that they're on the right track. It's become my number one piece of advice whenever I give a talk or help someone with their diet-related issues. I want to share this model with you as your springboard to healthier plant-based eating.

The VVPC plate

The VVPC plate has room for all types of plant-based food, and is the foundation of planning any meal, whether it's the occasional desk lunch, family dinner, or dining out at your favourite restaurant.

Whenever you eat lunch or dinner: imagine your plate split into four quarters. Fill two of these quarters with vegetables or salad, one with healthier carbs (page 51) and one with plant-based protein. Whenever you dish up or sit down to a meal, visualise this image, or just think of the letters VVPC.

SAVVY TIP

You can find a downloadable version to put on your fridge at azminanutrition.com

The size of dinner plates has grown over the past few decades. If you're watching your weight or rely on a lot of ultra-processed foods, choose a smaller plate. (I find that my dinner plate, which measures 25cm, gives me plenty of scope for nutritious, filling foods.) Otherwise, whole plant foods like beans, lentils, nuts, vegetables and wholegrains are such good foods that I believe it's generally fine for most people to use a regular dinner plate. In terms of how high you pile your food, there's no need to restrict whole vegetables that have been cooked healthily. When it comes to your carbohydrate or protein portion sizes, a good guide is the thickness of your palm.

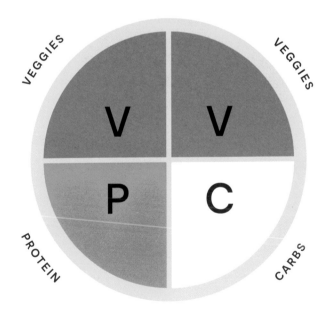

Remember that the VV portion is not only for vegetables, it's where your after-meal fruit fits, too.

RESEARCH ON PLATES

A plate like this forms an integral part of the advice given by the Glycemic Index Foundation[4], (a not-for-profit health promotion charity supported by The University of Sydney, Australia), primarily for people with diabetes and those watching their weight. The Oregon Health & Science University uses *My Heart-Healthy Plate*[5], a similar model intended to help prevent and manage heart disease, while the University of Massachusetts Medical School[6] also uses a similar diagram as a portion-controlling method for individuals with diabetes. As recently as mid-2019, the Government of Canada launched a version as their National Canada Food Guide[7] to help the whole population eat better and more sustainably. The Vegetarian Resource Group in Baltimore created a similar image in their *My Vegan Plate*[8]. In 2004, I introduced the *VVPC Picture Your Plate* as the basis of my best-selling book *Gi Plan*[9] as a simple way to help readers watch their weight and eat well.

Some of the plate models listed above single out calcium food sources outside of the plate. In my vegan VVPC plate, calcium is taken care of by the Nutrient Bridges (see page 7). My food swaps and meal ideas help you to bridge nutrient gaps and will set you on your way to a nutritionally well-rounded vegan diet.

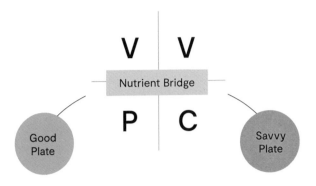

HOW DOES VVPC WORK WITH MIXED MEALS?

Veggies, carbs and protein sources won't always fit neatly onto each quarter of your plate, so you may find it tricky to assess which quarter should have which food on it. It's not a perfect science, so try to imagine the different food groups as best you can. After reading each chapter, you'll have more knowledge about vegetables, healthy carbohydrates and plant-based proteins, and this will help you when it comes to your VVPC plate.

THOUGHT LIFTER

Your imagination can be a powerful tool. Spending 20 seconds visualising the VVPC plate now will help you to remember it better when you're out and about.

VVPC IN PRACTICE

On the following pages I've worked out a few common dishes according to the VVPC plate to help you understand how to do it yourself.

Hummus and roast vegetable sandwich on wholegrain bread with a fruit smoothie

Vegetable noodles ready meal

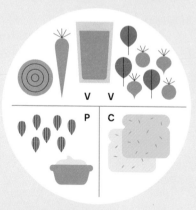

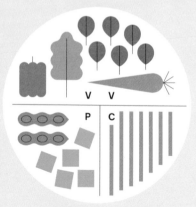

① Bread is your source of carbohydrates here, but obviously two slices aren't going to fit neatly onto a quarter of a plate! Use your judgement and keep in mind that two slices is a pretty standard portion size when it comes to bread.

② Hummus fills the protein requirement since it's made from chickpeas. Does the amount of hummus fill a quarter of your plate? If not, add some extra protein to your meal with a pot of edamame beans, a handful of nuts or swap the fruit smoothie for a soya-based alternative.

③ Here's where the VVPC plate really helps you get extra goodness from your meals: does the portion of roast veggies fill half the plate? Probably not, so add a side salad and a piece of fruit to fill out the portion.

① The noodles take care of your carbs quarter. You might find that some ready meals 'big up' the (cheaper) carbs and skimp on veggies or protein. Consider eating a bit less of the carbs, especially if they're refined and low in fibre.

② If there's tofu, edamame or other beans in the meal, they fit into the protein quarter. If there isn't enough, add a handful of cashews or some peas or sweetcorn.

③ As with the roast veggie sandwich, I doubt the ready meal provides enough veggies to cover half your plate. So, add a portion of stir-fried vegetables (there are packet versions ready to serve in minutes) or a generous handful of spinach.

Bean chilli and rice

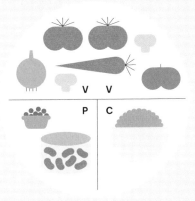

① Dish enough rice, ideally brown, to cover the carbs quarter of the plate.

② Beans provide carbohydrate and protein. Since you've already got the carbs covered, beans can be considered the protein in this meal — just make sure you've got enough of the beans and lentils, aside from the tomato and sauce, to fill the whole quarter. If you're eating a ready meal, you could add a can of sweetcorn or some peas to supplement the protein.

③ The two remaining quarters are for the two servings of vegetables, which in this case are the onions, tomatoes and other veggies you've added. If you haven't got enough vegetables to cover half your plate, add some salad on the side or end your meal with a piece of fruit.

THOUGHT LIFTER

The body knows when it needs to eat and when it's full, but over time we've become used to ignoring these signals. As you start to eat more consciously, you'll find it will become easier to listen to these signs.

You don't need to be this prescriptive about portions every day. Try to keep the VVPC plate in mind and ask yourself whether you've got close enough to the suggested portion sizes. Once you get used to seeing the way your VVPC plate looks and how you feel after eating a balanced meal this will become second nature.

If you need to lose weight or have type 2 diabetes, try the Zimbabwe hand jive method[10] for healthy portion sizes: protein portions should be around the thickness of your palm and a closed fist is an easy way to visualise the size of your carbs portion.

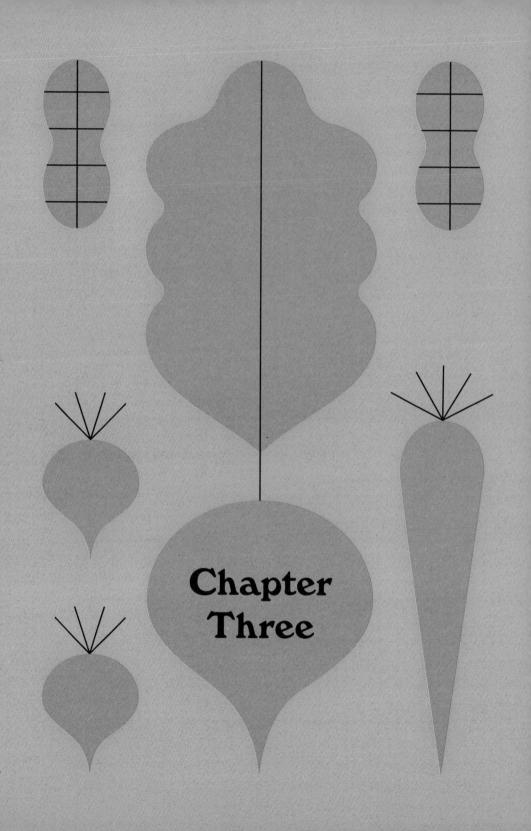

Chapter Three

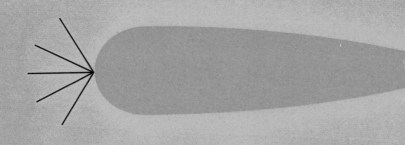

Vegetables:
The More
the Better

Vegetables:
The More the Better

Fruit and vegetables are nature's convenience food. Most are very easy to prepare and give you natural goodness in the form of fibre and a range of vitamins, minerals and phytochemicals (substances in plants that have been shown to have therapeutic benefits). They have no cholesterol, no added salt or added sugar. And some even come in their own plastic-free packaging, like satsumas, lychees and edamame.

How many fruits and vegetables should you be eating?

The World Health Organization (WHO) recommends that we should eat at least 400g fruit and vegetables a day. This equates to at least five 80–100g portions. Conveniently, most whole fruits are around this weight; an apple, a pear and an orange are 80–100g. Bear in mind there are two magic words in this recommendation that are often forgotten: 'at least'.

RESEARCH

Studies show that diets rich in fruit and vegetables are associated with lower risks of heart disease, strokes, obesity and some types of cancer, such as bowel cancer. A major review of ninety-five studies published in 2017 at Imperial College London found that 800g (equivalent to ten-a-day) of fruit and vegetables was associated with a significant reduction in these diseases as well as a 31% reduction in premature deaths.[11]

For most people, ten-a-day can feel like an ambitious goal, but the good news is that vegans are probably likely to be achieving much more than five-a-day. Eat a wide variety of different types of fruit and vegetables for your overall health, including a healthy gut.

Vegetables (as well as any fruit after your meal) make up half your VVPC plate. Some vegetables, like beans, peas, lentils and sweetcorn, are also protein-providers. If you're counting these vegetables as your protein, then enjoy a range of other vegetables and salad to fill the VV section.

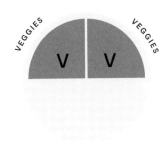

Choose fresh, frozen or canned veg in unsalted water. Try to have at least two different veggies to give your meal colour and a variety of nutrients, tastes and textures.

Sometimes you might not be able to fill half your plate with vegetables or salad. Since fruits offer similar nutrients, try to have some fruit for dessert but 'count it' as though it were filling one of the veggie quarters of your plate.

Natural goodness

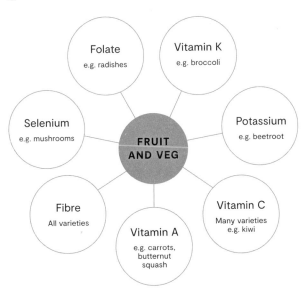

PECAN AND STRAWBERRY YOGURT

Stir 2 tbsp chopped pecans and some sliced strawberries into fruity dairy-free yogurt alternative.

NUTTY SNACK POT

Mix 2 tbsp of your favourite nuts with 3 chopped dried dates.

PURE WHITE

Fill the holes of canned lychees with blanched almonds or cashews and toss in desiccated coconut.

FRUIT BREAD

Toast a slice of raisin bread and top with blueberries and a dusting of icing sugar.

BANANA AND MELON PICK-ME-UP

Slice a banana and mix with cantaloupe melon cubes. Serve chilled with halved black grapes.

Fruit: friend or foe?

I'm often asked if fruit is 'still allowed', since there's been so much hype about the sugar in fruit and fruit juice. Fruit juice does not have the fibre that is intact in whole fruits. Although you get vitamin C from juice, it is also high in sugars, especially if you drink large amounts, which can damage your teeth. If you blend your own juice or smoothies at home, why not try adding some vegetables so you get less sugar? A glass of 150ml fruit juice counts once only as one of your five-a-day fruit and veg and is a sensible portion size. But, what's important for vegans is that the vitamin C from fruit juice can help you absorb the iron in meals (see page 80), so it is an important item on your shopping list. Enjoy fruit juice and smoothies with meals so long as you're keeping to the recommended amount of 30g 'free sugars' a day (see page 57). A glass of 150ml orange juice, whether fresh, chilled or UHT, has about 12g free sugars.

Fruit is full of good stuff like potassium that helps to regulate your blood pressure, and fibre that is essential for a healthy gut. Fruit also contains sugar, but this is natural sugar, not 'free sugars'. Although most fruits are roughly the same calories weight for weight, it might be easier to overeat fruits like mango, grapes and pineapple as they don't come in handy portion sizes, so go easy on these if you're watching your weight. Dried fruits are more concentrated in sugar and, weight for weight, are higher in calories than fresh fruit. But as you'll see from chapter 9, many are great providers of micronutrients. In the end, good nutrition is about having a wide variety of all types of fruit and vegetables.

What counts as a portion?

So many people are still confused about what counts as one portion of fruit or vegetables. Here are some examples (you'll find a more extensive list on azminanutrition.com):

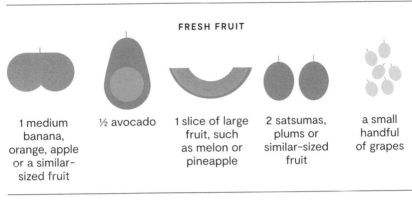

FRESH FRUIT

1 medium banana, orange, apple or a similar-sized fruit

½ avocado

1 slice of large fruit, such as melon or pineapple

2 satsumas, plums or similar-sized fruit

a small handful of grapes

DRIED FRUIT

1 heaped tbsp dried fruit, such as sultanas, currants or cranberries

2 prunes

3 dried dates

CANNED FRUITS AND VEGETABLES

| 6 apricot halves | 2 guava halves | 3 segments of green jackfruit | 3 heaped tbsp ackee |

JUICES (COUNT ONCE A DAY ONLY)

150ml unsweetened fresh fruit juice

150ml smoothie

150ml vegetable juice

VEGETABLES AND SALADS

1 medium carrot

3 heaped tbsp sweetcorn

8 cauliflower florets

4 heaped tbsp cooked kale or spinach

10 fingers of okra

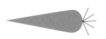

10 radishes

1 medium onion

1 cereal bowl of mixed salad

7 cherry tomatoes

5cm piece of cucumber

PULSES (COUNT ONCE A DAY ONLY BECAUSE THEY DON'T HAVE THE FULL RANGE OF NUTRIENTS FOUND IN OTHER VEGETABLES)

3 heaped tbsp beans, chickpeas, peas or lentils

VEGETABLES

The greater the variety of colours in the fruit and vegetables you eat, the wider the range of nutrients you'll get. Try to eat vegetables or fruit from each colour group over the course of a week to get wider nutritional benefits. Check out these colourful ways to spruce up your favourite vegetables:

RED BEETROOT DIP	Mix grated cooked beetroot with dairy-free yogurt alternative, a dash of lime juice, a sprinkling of garlic granules, chopped peanuts and freshly chopped parsley.
ORANGE VEG MEDLEY	Place layers of thinly sliced carrots, orange peppers, butternut squash and red onion onto a greased baking tray, flavouring with black pepper and fresh thyme between the layers. Drizzle with rapeseed oil and cover with about 100ml vegan stock. Bake for about 25 minutes at 200°C/gas mark 6 until the vegetables are tender.
PURPLE AUBERGINE BOATS	Cut an aubergine in half lengthways and remove most of the flesh, leaving you with a thin 'boat'. Roast the boats with some olive oil for about 20 minutes at 200°C/gas mark 6. Meanwhile, dice the scooped-out flesh and sauté with chopped onion and garlic until soft. Season lightly, add freshly chopped parsley and stuff the cooked boats with the aubergine and onion mix. Scatter with grated vegan mozzarella and grill until melted.
MUSHROOM MOUSSAKA	Make a moussaka using wild mushrooms instead of minced meat. They bring a yummy umami flavour, especially if you use dried porcini mushrooms that have been soaked in water to bring out the richness.
PINK RHUBARB SLAW	Mix finely sliced rhubarb with shredded carrots and white cabbage. Shake a little olive oil, maple syrup, lemon juice and black pepper in a jar and drizzle this dressing over the slaw.
GREEN MEAN BROCCOLI CUISINE	Stir-fry small florets of broccoli in a little rapeseed oil. Add a dash of soy sauce and chilli flakes to taste. Finish with a drizzle of sesame oil and toasted sesame seeds.

PLANT POWER

Vegan diets are perfectly placed to provide a range of powerful vitamins, minerals, antioxidants and fibre through eating a range of vegetables and fruit.

Chapter
Four

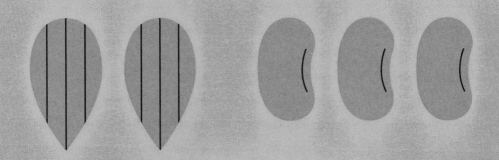

Kings
and Queens
of Protein

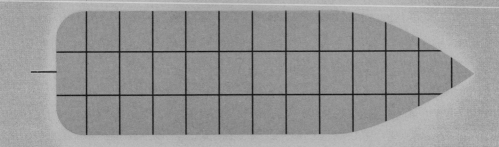

Benefits of protein

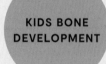

MUSCLE GROWTH

Contributes to a growth in muscle mass

HEALTHY BONES

Contributes to the maintenance of normal bones

SUPPORTS MUSCLE MASS

Contributes to the maintenance of muscle mass

KIDS BONE DEVELOPMENT

Needed for normal growth and development of bone in children

Kings and Queens of Protein

We need protein every day and there's no reason why a plant-based diet can't give you enough: you get protein from beans, lentils, peas, sweetcorn, nuts, soya, seeds, meat substitutes, dairy-free drinks, and so on. And you don't need to buy expensive protein powders to supplement your diet.

What does protein do?

Protein helps muscles grow and repair, it's needed for healthy bones and is crucial for bone development in children[12]. Protein also gives you energy – pure protein has the same number of calories as pure carbs – 4 kilocalories (kcal) per gram. I'd much rather you use protein for its important bone and muscle functions than as a source of energy, so you need to make sure you're eating enough food to allow protein to do its job. Plant protein, such as beans and lentils, will also help you achieve five-a-day fruit and vegetables, as well as boost fibre intake. And of course, plant proteins are broadly speaking more sustainable than animal proteins.

Why you need to think about protein

Many people I know who've become vegan think it's simply a matter of cutting out meat and eating vegetables instead. But they often forget that meat was providing their protein, so to replace that protein they need protein-rich vegetables (like peas, beans, lentils and sweetcorn), not just any varieties.

All proteins are made up of building blocks called amino acids. Nine of these are essential, which means that the body can't manufacture them and so we must get them from food. High-quality proteins contain all nine essential amino acids in adequate amounts. When part of a varied diet, plant proteins can provide enough essential amino acids; the key is to ensure you eat a variety throughout the day. Protein is also found in carbs such as wheat, rice and pasta, so consuming healthy combinations will help you get the full range of essential amino acids.

You don't need to eat different plant proteins at the same meal to give you good-quality protein, but you may find you do this anyway.

THOUGHT LIFTER

'One cannot think well, love well, sleep well, if one has not dined well.'

— Virginia Woolf, *A Room of One's Own*

DIGESTIBILITY

Protein from meat and dairy is typically more digestible than protein from whole plant foods such as beans. Many plant proteins such as tofu and mycoprotein still have good digestibilty.

PROTEIN QUALITY

Animal proteins generally have a wide range of essential and non-essential amino acids, which are the building blocks of proteins. Plant-based proteins vary – some, such as hemp seeds, will have all nine essential amino acids, but others may not and this affects their protein quality.

PICKING YOUR PROTEINS

TYPE OF PROTEIN

Soya-based drinks and tofu contain all nine essential amino acids and the protein is of a high digestibility too. The protein quality of peas and kidney beans is almost as good as soya, so enjoy them regularly.

VARY AND MIX

Eat a good range of healthy foods to get the most power from your plant protein. You probably do this naturally: beans on toast, cereal with plant-based drinks or lentils with rice. You don't need to have different types of protein at the same meal, just throughout the day.

Your daily protein requirements depend on your weight (0.75g protein per kg bodyweight), so if you weigh 60kg, this equates to 45g protein per day. We all vary in our needs, but on average, adult men need about 55g protein and women 45g (on food labels you will see this as a Reference Intake (RI) of 50g). Some expert dietitians who specialise in vegan diets[13] believe that vegans need more protein than meat-eaters, because many plant foods like beans and lentils don't seem to be as well digested as proteins from meat and dairy. The American Academy of Nutrition and Dietetics recommends that vegans should aim for 1.1g protein per kg of body weight[14]. So, if you weigh 60kg, this would equate to 66g a day.

I advise most of my vegan patients to aim for about 20g of protein at each of their three meals, and a small amount of protein at snack time if they like, which is a little more than what's currently recommended for the average population. This is especially the case in people who are sporty (you need protein for muscle recovery) or over sixty years old (your muscles can start to become weaker and waste as you get older). This is to compensate for the lower digestibility of plant proteins, such as beans and legumes. If most of your protein comes from tofu or meat substitutes made from soya protein or mycoprotein (sold as Quorn™), digestibility isn't a problem.

Food labelling RI for calories and other nutrients

Energy	8400kj/2000kcal
Total fat	70g
Saturates	20g
Sugars	90g
Protein	50g
Salt	6g

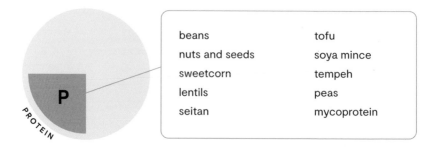

beans	tofu
nuts and seeds	soya mince
sweetcorn	tempeh
lentils	peas
seitan	mycoprotein

The protein section makes up about a quarter of your VVPC plate. In flexitarian diets, this is where chicken, meat or fish would sit. In vegan diets, many protein foods like beans and pulses are also vegetables, so they could sit in the veg half too. To get nutritional balance, I suggest you place only high-protein vegetables in the protein quarter of your plate.

Protein type

Protein quality is important when it comes to maintaining muscle mass. A varied vegan diet can give you all the essential amino acids you need, but bear in mind that some plant foods won't give you enough of the full range of amino acids. Foods with fewer essential amino acids are considered to be lower quality protein. For example, two particular amino acids called lysine and (to a lesser extent) methionine, have been found to be typically lower in many plant-based foods – more on this below.

High-quality proteins include soya, mycoprotein[15] (sold as Quorn™), chickpeas, beans, lentils, hemp seeds and nuts. Make sure you always have a protein source at every meal. Eating soups and salads oozing with colourful vegetables might sound virtuous, but they won't necessarily give you enough protein.

VARY AND MIX

Grains like wheat and rice are relatively low in the amino acid lysine but do provide methionine. Beans and peas are relatively high in lysine, yet they're lower in methionine[16]. So, eating a variety of plant-based foods helps you get the best amino acid combination. If you really don't like beans and lentils, you can get lysine from tempeh, soya meat substitutes, seitan and to a lesser extent from carbs such as quinoa and amaranth[17]; ideally try to have legumes regularly as they are a rich source.

KINGS AND
QUEENS
OF PROTEIN

CEREAL GRAINS

Higher in methionine

Lower in lysine

BEANS AND PULSES

Higher in lysine

Lower in methionine

Because most plant foods will give you some methionine, it's the lysine that's a particularly important amino acid for vegans. So, make sure you eat foods that supply this Nutrient Bridge.

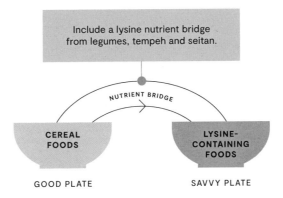

Include a lysine nutrient bridge from legumes, tempeh and seitan.

NUTRIENT BRIDGE

CEREAL FOODS

LYSINE-CONTAINING FOODS

GOOD PLATE

SAVVY PLATE

Whole plant foods are generally great natural sources of fibre, vitamins, minerals, healthy fats and antioxidants. They're also typically low in saturated fat, sodium and cholesterol. This may be part of the reason why studies suggest associations between vegetarian and vegan diets and lower risk of certain diseases, such as heart disease and type 2 diabetes.

Your meatless protein guide

If protein makes up 12% of the calories of any given food, that food is legally considered to be a significant source of protein. For simplicity, I've created a handy guide to help you get enough protein at every meal. Each food in the list overleaf will give you 5g protein and I suggest you aim for around 20g protein per meal (see page 37). Some of these tasty ideas are so rich in protein that you could get your 5g by eating just a small amount – simply double the quantity to give you 10g protein per serving.

Breakfast cereals, breads and many other carbs also provide protein – remember that carbs belong in another section of your VVPC plate (see page 19), though they do count towards your daily protein intake.

How to get 5g protein[18]

Oat, almond, hemp and coconut milk alternatives, as well as vegan cheese alternatives, currently have too little protein to be included in this list.

MEAT AND DAIRY SUBSTITUTES

25g tempeh

65g steamed tofu

20g fried tofu

90g (2–3 tbsp) soya Greek yogurt alternative

150ml (small glass) soya drink

7g seitan (wheat gluten) meat substitute

½ Quorn™-based vegan sausage roll (e.g. Greggs)

½ vegan Quorn™ fillet (35g)

BEANS AND PULSES

90g (3–4 tbsp) peas

100g (¼ large can) baked beans

65g (2 tbsp) boiled mung dhal

60g (2 tbsp) boiled red lentils

60g (¼ large can) red kidney beans, drained

75g (3 tbsp) chickpeas or hummus

70g (3 tbsp) refried beans

45g (2–3 tbsp) edamame beans

NUTS AND SEEDS

25g (2 tbsp) sunflower seeds

30g (3–4 tbsp) chia seeds

20g (2 tbsp) pumpkin seeds

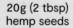
20g (2 tbsp) hemp seeds

KINGS AND QUEENS OF PROTEIN

| 30g (3 tbsp) flaxseeds | 35g (about a handful) walnuts | 25g (about a handful) almonds | 22g (3 tsp) peanut butter | 20g (a small handful) peanuts |

GRAINS

| 100g cooked quinoa | 140g boiled wholegrain rice | 70g cooked couscous |

| 90g (1 cupped handful) cooked pasta) | 45g (3 tbsp) raw porridge oats | 60g (2) oatcakes |

BREADS AND POTATOES

| 55g (1 large slice) wholegrain bread | 50g (1) wholegrain pitta | 44g (1 slice) soya and linseed bread | 220g (1 large) baked potato |

Soya – good or bad?

You may have seen headlines linking soya to breast cancer or interference with male hormones. Many of the studies are based on animals and the evidence is weak.

Soya has long been recognised as a meat and dairy substitute although there still appears to be confusion about its potential effects on health. Benefits on heart health have been linked to compounds called isoflavones that appear to act like oestrogen. Most media headlines have tended to focus on whether soya consumption can influence sex and thyroid hormones[19]. In reality, however, it has been reported that this is unlikely given that most vegetarians and vegans seem to have relatively low isoflavone intakes – especially if they are eating a variety of foods[20].

RESEARCH

An extensive review of soya health benefits and risks was conducted in 2014[20]. The authors concluded that eating moderate amounts of less processed soya foods may offer modest health benefits. This also helps to minimise potentially negative effects on health. They acknowledge that we currently don't have enough research to understand the long-term health effects of a diet rich in processed 'modern soya foods'.

Official dietary guidance remains to be developed in relation to soya and its constituent isoflavones, but I encourage people to eat soya as a meat and dairy substitute because it is a highly digestible, high-quality protein and an essential component of a varied vegan diet. Foods such as soya and edamame beans, tofu, tempeh and roasted soya nuts can make a positive nutritional contribution to your diet. If you opt for more processed versions, such as sausages made from soya-based meat substitute or burgers made from wheat protein, eat them in moderation, just like with any highly processed foods, and as part of a balanced and varied diet.

When you're not eating as much meat and dairy as you used to, you might be taking in fewer calories. For some people, getting enough calories on a vegan diet can be a challenge, as plant foods tend to be bulkier and higher in fibre, so you can feel fuller quicker and find it difficult to eat enough.

If this resonates with you, don't be afraid to increase the number of meals you have, especially if you're physically active. My sporty vegan daughter found that she was getting so full after each meal that she couldn't finish it, but then she'd get hungry again a couple of hours later. So, she decided to either separate her meals out into two halves, or listen to her body and eat another light meal when she got hungry again. If your plate is filled with nutritious plant-based foods and you're still hungry after your meal, there's no problem having more of the good stuff. Just don't use it as an excuse to overeat or fill up on ultra-processed or fast foods!

Not being able to manage enough calories for your body's needs can be a concern, particularly if you're athletic, as you'll be burning calories during exercise. If you're taking in fewer calories than you need for daily activities, your body will start to use dietary protein as fuel (energy), so all the protein you eat won't be available for muscle recovery and repair – seems like a waste of good protein to me.

According to the evidence-based resource VeganHealth.org, if you're not eating enough calories to keep your weight steady, you should aim to eat more high-protein foods[21].

If you want to lose weight, you still need to be thinking about getting goodness out of your calories so that you stay healthy in the long term. That's why there's a quarter of your VVPC plate dedicated to protein, each meal, every day. Chapter 9 on micronutrients as well as the Nutrient Bridges in this book are my suggestions to help you get more value from your calories.

THOUGHT LIFTER

If this all feels complicated as you're reading it, don't worry. I've been a student of nutrition for three decades and I'm still learning. Trust that whatever information you retain is enough for now and you can always come back to it another time.

SAVVY TIP

Potatoes aren't usually thought of as a good source of protein, but you can get almost 5g from a large baked potato. Add ½ large can of baked beans and a generous sprinkling of pumpkin seeds and you've reached 20g protein for lunch!

Five more protein nutrient bridges

GOOD PLATE		NUTRIENT BRIDGE		SAVVY PLATE
Salad	+	A handful of nuts	=	✓
Stir-fry	+	2 tbsp seeds	=	✓
Takeaway meal	+	Peas, baked beans or edamame	=	✓
Nachos with salsa	+	Soya Greek yogurt alternative	=	✓
Toast	+	Nut butter	=	✓

Protein Nutrient Bridges like tofu, which is a high-quality plant protein, can help you create balanced meals. But some people struggle with tofu as they find it tasteless. Check out my simple ideas to bring tofu to life:

CREAMY PASTA SAUCE

Sauté garlic and onion in a little olive oil. Blitz silken tofu with the cooked garlic and onion, lemon juice, vegan stock and B12-enriched nutritional yeast. Cook to a creamy consistency, adding some plant-based drink if you prefer a thinner sauce. Flavour with fresh thyme, oregano and seasoning and smother over your favourite wholegrain pasta.

TANDOORI TOFU

Marinate firm tofu chunks in a mix of tandoori powder or paste, tomato purée and a little dairy-free yogurt alternative. Grill until charred and top with coriander leaves. Delicious stuffed into wholewheat pitta bread with shredded crispy lettuce.

FAJITA FILLER

Lightly toss firm tofu strips in fajita seasoning and grill or shallow-fry until cooked. Lay onto warmed tortilla wraps with stir-fried onion, thinly sliced peppers and guacamole. Roll into wraps and serve with tomato salsa.

THOUGHT LIFTER

Celebrate every success. Taking on one tip is one more than yesterday.

Shopping for protein

PANTRY ESSENTIALS

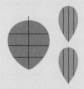

Nuts (all types)

Seeds (all types)

Canned beans
(all types)

Canned
chickpeas

Canned
sweetcorn

Dried beans
and lentils

Nut butters

FRIDGE AND FREEZER ESSENTIALS

Tofu (any type)

Soya-based
meat substitutes

Mycoprotein
(sold as Quorn™)

Tempeh

Seitan

Soya drink

Soya yogurt
alternative

Frozen peas

Frozen
edamame beans

Frozen
sweetcorn

Hummus

Sesame tahini

Your protein checklist

☐ Make sure you have a source of protein at every meal – aim for 20g.

☐ Vary your protein throughout the day – mix and match so you get good-quality protein with a wide range of amino acids every day.

☐ Don't assume all vegan foods are nutritious. Compare labels and choose plant-based foods that give you enough protein.

☐ Regularly enjoy high-quality proteins like tofu, soya-based meats, mycoprotein, peas or kidney beans.

☐ Choose a soya-based dairy alternative if you can, as it typically has more protein than other plant-based drinks.

PLANT POWER

A vegan diet can supply a full range of essential amino acids by mixing different types of protein foods in a day. Simply eat enough protein to overcome reduced digestibility from whole plant proteins.

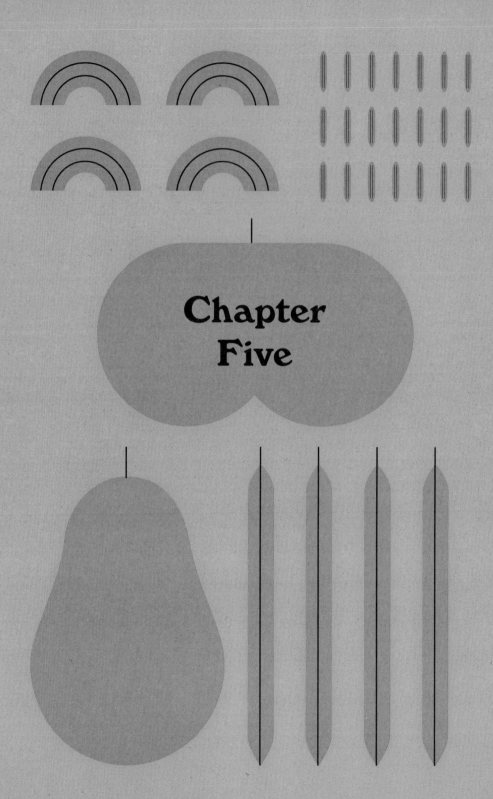

Chapter Five

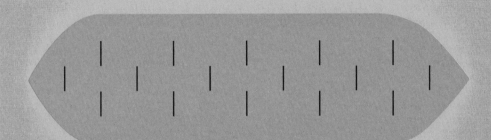

Here's Looking at You, Carb

Here's Looking at You, Carb

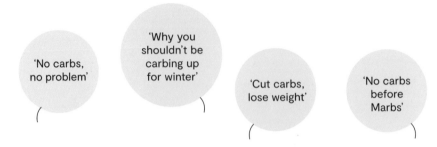

'No carbs, no problem'

'Why you shouldn't be carbing up for winter'

'Cut carbs, lose weight'

'No carbs before Marbs'

Carbs: not the villain they're made out to be

We're all used to seeing sensational headlines like these in the press. It's a common misconception that starchy foods are the culprit for weight gain, but gram for gram they actually contain less than half the calories of fat. With all the conflicting information out there, it can be tough to know whether to ditch the carbs or embrace them with a clear conscience.

What do carbohydrates do?

Carbohydrates are fuel for the body; when digested, they're broken down into molecules of glucose, which is the primary fuel for your brain and muscles. Some starchy carbs like wholegrain breakfast cereals provide fibre, B vitamins or minerals such as iron and calcium. It's important to remember that the amount of carbs you eat is less important than the type — quality matters.

Not all carbs are created equal

Brown rice and biscuits are both carbs, but they definitely don't provide the same calories or nutrients. Just like fats and proteins, not all carbohydrates are the same. There are different ways to define carbohydrate foods. One way is to divide them into carbs that are predominantly made of starch and carbs that are high sugar-providers. For good health, most of your carbs should come from higher fibre sources like wholegrains and most of your sugars should come from natural sources like fruit and vegetables.

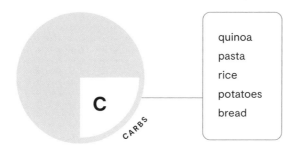

quinoa
pasta
rice
potatoes
bread

Approximately half of your daily calories should come from starchy foods and carbohydrates make up about a quarter of your VVPC plate. People with type 2 diabetes who need to lose weight may benefit from carbohydrate restriction (less than 130g a day) to help manage blood glucose levels more effectively; speak to your healthcare professional if you need guidance on this.

Choose high-fibre options like brown rice and pasta, potatoes in their skins or wholegrain bread. Sweet potatoes are mainly made up of carbohydrate and are higher in fibre than regular potatoes. In terms of your VVPC plate, they sit in the carbs section because they are a starchy vegetable, albeit with extra nutrition.

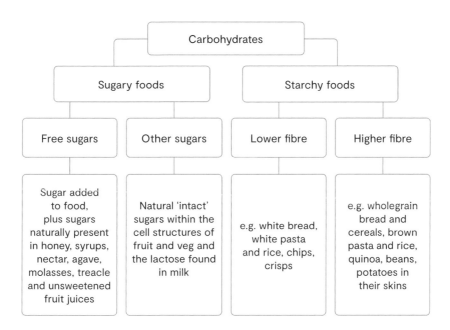

Carbohydrates

Sugary foods — Starchy foods

Free sugars | Other sugars | Lower fibre | Higher fibre

Sugar added to food, plus sugars naturally present in honey, syrups, nectar, agave, molasses, treacle and unsweetened fruit juices

Natural 'intact' sugars within the cell structures of fruit and veg and the lactose found in milk

e.g. white bread, white pasta and rice, chips, crisps

e.g. wholegrain bread and cereals, brown pasta and rice, quinoa, beans, potatoes in their skins

Benefits of fibre

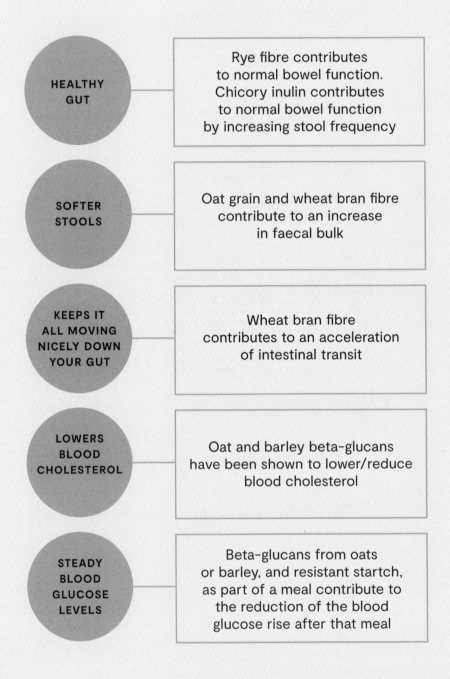

HEALTHY GUT

Rye fibre contributes
to normal bowel function.
Chicory inulin contributes
to normal bowel function
by increasing stool frequency

SOFTER STOOLS

Oat grain and wheat bran fibre
contribute to an increase
in faecal bulk

KEEPS IT ALL MOVING NICELY DOWN YOUR GUT

Wheat bran fibre
contributes to an acceleration
of intestinal transit

LOWERS BLOOD CHOLESTEROL

Oat and barley beta-glucans
have been shown to lower/reduce
blood cholesterol

STEADY BLOOD GLUCOSE LEVELS

Beta-glucans from oats
or barley, and resistant starch,
as part of a meal contribute to
the reduction of the blood
glucose rise after that meal

Beans and lentils contain carbs and protein, so they fall into the protein quarter of your plate if you're also eating a source of carbohydrate such as rice. If you're eating a low-carb protein like tofu or mycoprotein that occupies the protein quarter, then beans, peas, sweetcorn or lentils could make up the carbs or even veggie portion of your plate. Remember in both examples, filling half your plate with a variety of vegetables, salad and a piece of fruit brings you closer to a beautifully balanced meal.

Fibre and carbs: what's the connection and why do we need fibre?[22]

Fibre is the part of plant foods that can't be completely broken down by your digestive enzymes. High-fibre foods like wholegrain cereals can help to regulate bowel habits and prevent uncomfortable symptoms like constipation. The type of fibre found in fruit and vegetables goes through a process of fermentation in your digestive system, which may contribute to heathy gut bacteria.[23]

Rye fibre can have a favourable effect on your gut only when you eat foods that are labelled 'high (or rich) in rye fibre'. More and more manufacturers are adding inulin to foods to increase the fibre and so that they can claim advantages to gut health. You get this beneficial effect of inulin when you eat 12g chicory inulin. Wheat bran fibre, inulin and beta-glucans are usually declared on a food label.

FIBRE AND HEALTH

In 2015, the UK Scientific Advisory Committee on Nutrition (SACN) conducted a thorough scientific review of the links between carbohydrates and health[24]. Here are some of their findings:

1. A high-fibre diet is associated with a reduced incidence of heart disease, strokes, obesity and type 2 diabetes.
2. High-fibre diets rich in cereals, fruits and vegetables can lead to increased faecal weight (bulkier stools, since fibre acts like a sponge and holds a lot of water) and decreased intestinal transit time (meaning food moves through the intestine in less time). A shorter transit time is healthier.
3. Higher consumption of fibre is associated with reduced incidence of colorectal cancer.

SACN recommends we should aim to eat 30g fibre every day. You can't get fibre from animal products, so vegan diets tend to offer plenty of fibre. What you need to be aware of in terms of overall dietary balance, is that substances called phytates found in some plant-based foods, such as wheat bran and dried beans, can reduce the absorption of other nutrients, including calcium, iron and zinc (more on this in later chapters, see page 105). These foods are great fibre-providers – just don't rely on them for your micronutrients.

When I analysed my sample menu plans, I found that it's actually easy to get more than the daily recommended 30g fibre on a varied plant-based diet. When you eat more fibre than you used to, you're likely to have a change in bowel habits, for example, you might have a greater urgency to 'go'. This should improve once your body adjusts – these changes can be seen as reassurance that you're on the right track!

SAVVY TIP

When you eat more fibre, it's crucial that you also drink enough fluids to let the fibre work its magic. The British Dietetic Association recommends drinking 8–10 glasses of fluid a day at regular intervals when you consume more fibre.[25]

But not all vegan diets are high in fibre — it all depends on the types of foods you're eating. Strictly speaking, you could be filling up on fast foods, white-bread 'cheesey-style' sandwiches, crisps and takeaways and still be vegan. If this sounds like you, start thinking about small, manageable changes that you can make to increase your fibre intake.

A good long-term target is to make at least half of your grains wholegrain – so perhaps chop and change between wholegrain and white pasta if eating brown pasta regularly is a step too far. There are also 50/50 pastas and breads that can help you to eat more wholegrains without switching completely. You can do the same with wholegrain cereals, rice, breads and so on. Look for 'source of fibre' or 'high in fibre' on food packaging to help you choose higher fibre options. This legal terminology means the product is certified as being a source of fibre.

Five ways
to up your fibre

1. Starchy foods e.g. wholegrain breads and breakfast cereals, brown rice, quinoa, brown pasta, potatoes in their skins, porridge and muesli.

2. Legumes e.g. beans, lentils, peas, sweetcorn, baked beans, chickpeas and hummus.

3. Vegetables e.g. carrots, sweet potatoes, green beans, broccoli and kale.

4. Fruits e.g. apples, pears, peaches, satsumas, grapes, bananas and pineapple.

5. Nuts, nut butters and seeds.

ONE STEP AT A TIME...

LOW FIBRE	BETTER	EVEN BETTER	BEST
1 slice of white bread with butter and jam	1 slice of white bread with peanut butter	1 slice of whole-meal bread with peanut butter	1 slice of wholemeal bread with peanut butter and ½ small banana
1.4g fibre; 11g (added) sugar	2.1g fibre; 2.0g (added) sugar	3.9g fibre; 2.0g (added) sugar	5.0g fibre; 9g (mainly natural) sugar

There's some evidence that fibre-filled foods can leave us feeling fuller for longer[26].

GOOD PLATE		NUTRIENT BRIDGE		SAVVY PLATE
Cornflakes	+	Mix in a few bran flakes for the first week and gradually progress to eating more bran flakes than cornflakes. Add a handful of sliced almonds for added calcium	=	✓
'Buttered' toast	+	Move from white bread to half and half, and then to wholegrain bread only. Or stick with white bread (it's a source of calcium) and sprinkle some seeds on top of your spread for a fibre boost	=	✓
Takeaway vegetable chow mein	+	Add some extra vegetables like sweetcorn or peas, which will also give you extra protein	=	✓
Baked potato with vegan cheese alternative	+	Eat the skin and top with added fibre in the form of baked beans or coleslaw	=	✓
Hummus	+	Mix in diced red onion and peppers	=	✓

High-fibre wholegrains are the better type of carbohydrate but that doesn't mean you can only eat 'brown foods'. Mix and match to find what works for you.

Is sugar the enemy of good health?

Contrary to what you may read, sugar alone is not responsible for the obesity epidemic; a whole host of factors, including our sedentary lifestyles, high-calorie foods and drinks, and large portion sizes are also to blame. The indesputable fact about sugar and health is that drinking large amounts of sugar-rich drinks, especially in between meals can increase your risk of tooth decay.

Sugar-rich foods and drinks tend to be high in calories. As a nation, we need to be cutting our calories, so eating fewer sugar-rich cakes, biscuits, confectionery, sugar-sweetened drinks, and so on, is a good idea.

It's fine to have some sugar in your diet, but as with fibre, there are different types. The Reference Intake (RI) for total sugars is 90g a day, which includes 30g 'free sugars' (around 7 sugar cubes). Foods high in free sugars, such as sweets and sugar-sweetened drinks, are typically digested more quickly (often called high glycaemic index or high GI foods), which can cause spikes in blood sugar levels and do not offer the health benefits associated with food made up predominantly of sugars found in fruit and milk.

Food labels in the UK currently display total sugar content only, so you can't tell how much of the sugar is free sugars. It can be helpful to compare the total sugar content of different brands and choose the lower sugar option.

SAVVY TIP

A typical 330ml can of cola can contain as much as 30g free sugars (that's your limit for the day), while a fruit such as an apple, pears or orange has an average of 10g intact sugars, which is about a sixth of your recommended daily limit.

I've seen media stories focusing heavily on the 'hidden sugar' in nutrient-dense foods such as wholegrain breakfast cereals, fruit and vegetable smoothies, peanut butter and pasta sauces. I believe we should be supporting people to make healthier choices, and to cut down on unhealthy energy-dense foods like cakes, biscuits, and sugar-sweetened drinks. There is a place for all foods; healthy eating is about balance, enjoyment and portion control.

THOUGHT LIFTER

If you're craving chocolate, have a handful or raisins or dates, set a timer for 10 minutes, then see if that craving is still there. If plain dates don't inspire you, try dolloping on some peanut butter, sprinkling over a couple of cacao nibs or topping with a raspberry.

At the end of the day, it's all about balance! Enjoy your food, savour a wide range of fruit and vegetables, eat more fibre, less saturated fat, sugar and salt, and allow yourself small amounts of whatever sugary foods you really enjoy.

Total sugars
No more than 90g a day

Free sugars
(includes added sugars)

Other sugars

Sugar added
to food, and
sugars naturally
present
in honey,
syrups and
unsweetened
fruit juices

Adults should
consume
no more than
30g sugar
(7 sugar cubes)
a day

Stucturally
intact fructose
found in fruit
and vegetables.
Lactose found
in dairy foods.

Total sugars
minus free
sugars leaves
you with 60g
of other sugars
a day

PLANT POWER

The takeaway: carbs are not the enemy! Many types are an essential part of a varied diet. Vegan diets can be a cut above the rest when it comes to fibre.

Your carbohydrate checklist

☐ Choose high-fibre carbs like brown rice and pasta in preference to refined or white varieties.

☐ Eat more whole plant carbohydrate foods such as beans, lentils, quinoa and whole grains.

☐ Aim for 30g fibre every day.

☐ Drink 8–10 glasses of fluid daily when you increase your fibre intake.

☐ Compare labels and opt for products that are lower in sugar.

☐ The sugars found in fruit (whole, canned in water, frozen or dried) are not free sugars, but the sugars in fruit juice *are* considered free sugars since the sugar is no longer within the fruit itself. So, although fruit juice provides nutrients, stick to 150ml servings to limit your free sugar and calorie intake. Try to drink these with a meal to reduce the effect of sugar on your teeth.

☐ You won't see 'free sugar' on nutrition labels, but it's there under different guises. Look out for ingredients like glucose, honey, molasses, palm sugar, syrup, dextrose, natural brown sugar and treacle — these are all free sugars. Popular syrups that are often touted as healthier versions of sugar like agave and maple syrup are also sources of free sugars.

☐ Consider the whole food, not just the sugar content. While they may contain some sugar, foods like peanut butter bring fibre and essential fats; fruit smoothies provide vitamin C, potassium and fibre; and fortified breakfast cereals provide B vitamins and iron.

☐ Cut down on obviously sugary foods, like sweetened drinks and cola, sweets, cakes, biscuits, chocolates, sweet pastries and desserts.

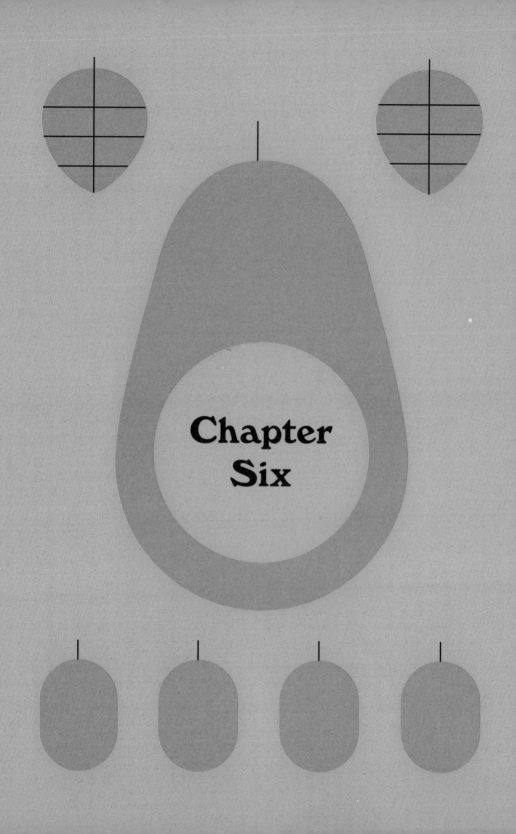

Chapter
Six

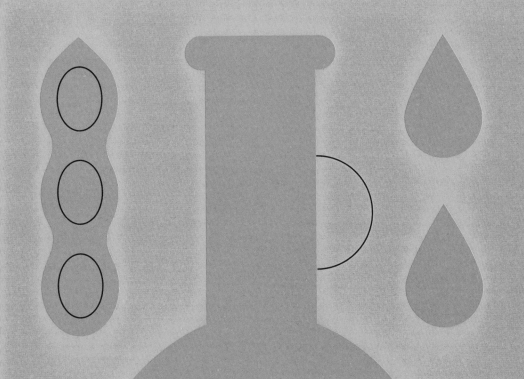

Getting Your Fats Straight

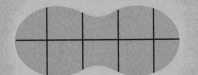
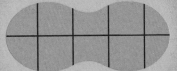

Getting Your Fats Straight

Why do we need fats?

Fats have been hotly debated for years and low-fat weight-loss diets often cast fat as the villain. I don't believe that's the case. Along with carbohydrates and protein, fats provide the calories we need for energy. We need fat for bodily processes, such as cell growth and hormone production, as well as insulation to protect our organs. Fat is also crucial for the absorption of fat-soluble vitamins from food, like vitamins A, D and E. Weight for weight, fat has over twice the calories of carbs and proteins (which is why many weight-loss programmes recommend a low-fat diet).

Fats are found in animal products like meat, fish, eggs and dairy, and in plant foods like oils, nuts, seeds and some fruits. Full-fat animal products are typically high in cholesterol-raising saturated fats, which are a risk factor in the development of heart disease[27].

RESEARCH: MORE PLANTS, LESS RISK

A meta-analysis[28] of forty studies published between 1960 and 2018 found that vegans had lower calorie and saturated fat intakes, lower BMI (body mass index), lower waist circumference and less low-density lipoprotein cholesterol (LDL), the so-called 'bad' cholesterol, in the bloodstream. The authors concluded that in most countries, a vegan diet was associated with fewer risk factors for heart disease.

The rise in vegan junk food means that plant-based foods may not always be filled with healthy fats. Whilst scanning supermarket shelves for dairy-free cheese alternatives and ready meals, I've noticed that many vegan foods use high levels of coconut oil, often misrepresented as a *better-for-you* fat (see page 68).

Most fat-containing foods have a combination of different types of fatty acids and sometimes one particular type is present in larger amounts. Animal fats tend to have more saturated fatty acids than plant-derived fats, while many (but not all) plant-based foods are mainly made up of mono- and poly-unsaturated fats and include most vegetable oils.

Polyunsaturated fats can be further split into different types of fatty acids, the two major ones are omega-3 and omega-6.

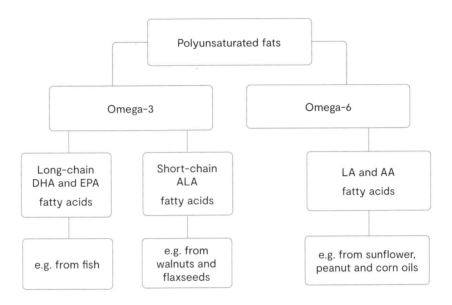

Most plant-based diets include enough omega-6 fatty acids from vegetable oils, nuts and seeds, but you do need to ensure you're getting adequate omega-3 fatty acids without animal foods.

WHAT DO OMEGA-3 FATTY ACIDS DO[29]?

Omega-3 polyunsaturated fatty acids include short-chain a-linolenic acid (ALA), long-chain eicosapentaenoic acid (EPA) and long-chain docosahexaenoic acid (DHA).

The richest source of EPA and DHA is oily fish; there are no plant-based food sources of EPA and DHA[30] but the body *is* able to convert ALA, found in plant-based foods like walnuts, flaxseeds (linseeds), hemp seeds and chia seeds into EPA and DHA — though this process can be slow and inefficient[31]. We can also get ALA from cooking oils such as rapeseed, flaxseed and hemp oil, and the body can convert them, albeit slowly, into EPA and DHA, so they can be useful foods in a vegan diet.

Plant-based omega-3 fatty acids aren't thought to have the same heart-protecting benefits as the omega-3 found in oily fish. We need both omega-3 and omega-6 fatty acids and it's likely that you'll be getting more than enough omega-6 from the abundance of fatty acids, such as linoleic acid (LA), in vegan foods like sunflower oil, nuts and seeds. This might sound good, but too much omega-6 in the form of LA can prevent the efficient conversion of ALA into EPA and DHA[32]. In short, eating a diet too rich in omega-6 (LA) could result in reduced blood levels of beneficial long-chain omega-3, even if you're including heaps of ALA (omega-3) in your diet.

According to The Vegan Society,[33] it's better to use rapeseed oil (which is rich in ALA) than sunflower, corn or sesame oils (all of which are high in LA), and they also suggest you avoid eating large amounts of sunflower and pumpkin seeds, as these are both high in LA.

SAVVY TIP

Rapeseed oil has around ten times more omega-3 than olive oil.

I recommend rapeseed oil for cooking, as it has a higher smoke point than olive oil. Oils start to degrade once they reach their smoke point, which means they are unsuitable for cooking at high temperatures or deep frying. You can usually find inexpensive bottles of rapeseed oil labelled as 'vegetable oil' in the supermarket. Simply look at the back of the bottle to check if it's made from 100% rapeseed oil. If you want to buy more expensive cold-pressed rapeseed oil, go ahead, but I find the regular type works just fine.

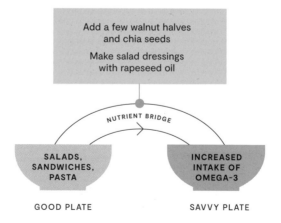

Add a few walnut halves and chia seeds

Make salad dressings with rapeseed oil

NUTRIENT BRIDGE

SALADS, SANDWICHES, PASTA

INCREASED INTAKE OF OMEGA-3

GOOD PLATE

SAVVY PLATE

GETTING YOUR FATS STRAIGHT

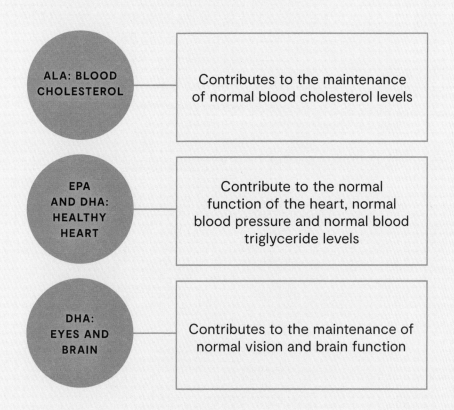

The European Food Safety Authority (EFSA) currently advises a dietary reference value (how much you should aim for each day) of 250mg EPA and DHA[34]. EFSA also suggests that an adequate intake of ALA is 0.5% of daily calories[35] (10kcal if you're having 2000kcal per day), which equates to 1.1g ALA per day, but this recommendation is not specifically for vegans so it assumes EPA and DHA would also be eaten. Hence, you probably need more than this on a vegan diet. The US Department of Health and Human Services recommends an Acceptable Intake (AI) of 1.6g ALA for men and 1.1g ALA for women[36].

It's been proposed that vegans need their own essential fatty acid diet guidelines[37]. While we don't yet have a set of dietary recommendations specifically for vegans (which could help take the conversion factors into account), you may want to stick with the EFSA's recommended intake and consider a vegan supplement like microalgae to provide sufficient EPA and DHA. Just keep in mind the daily recommendation of 250mg – a much higher dose doesn't mean a better supplement.

PLANT-BASED SOURCES OF OMEGA-3

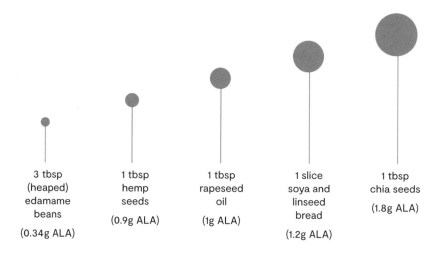

| 3 tbsp (heaped) edamame beans (0.34g ALA) | 1 tbsp hemp seeds (0.9g ALA) | 1 tbsp rapeseed oil (1g ALA) | 1 slice soya and linseed bread (1.2g ALA) | 1 tbsp chia seeds (1.8g ALA) |

When it comes to long-term health, you probably know that some fats are better than others. Foods high in trans fats can increase 'bad' LDL cholesterol and decrease the more protective HDL cholesterol in your blood. Trans fats used to be more of a concern, but since food manufacturers have largely cut them out, they're less of a problem nowadays. What's far more important is reducing your saturated fat intake.

RESEARCH

In 2018, SACN published a report on saturated fats and health[38] based on results from forty-seven systematic reviews and meta-analyses. The authors found that consuming high quantities of saturated fat is linked to raised blood cholesterol and is therefore associated with increased risk of heart disease. They concluded that no more than 10% of our daily calories should come from saturated fat. Public Health England, the British Heart Foundation and other leading organisations recommend that saturated fats be replaced with unsaturated fats.

Cholesterol isn't actually a fat, it's a sterol. It's present in a diet containing animal products, but your body also produces its own cholesterol as it's needed for bodily functions such as building cell membranes. Only around 15% of the cholesterol in your body comes from food, and the cholesterol in your diet has a limited impact on your blood cholesterol.[39,40]

PLANT POWER

Cholesterol is found in animal products such as eggs, shellfish, meat and dairy products so vegans have no cholesterol in their diets.

Coconut oil is having a real moment on the health and wellness stage. Whether you follow celebrity chefs, clean-eating gurus or fitness influencers on social media, it's hard to ignore the hype around all things coconut. I have no problem with fresh coconut or coconut water, but — believe it or not — coconut oil is actually devoid of the fibre, protein and carbohydrates that make fresh coconut so good for you. It might sound controversial, but I believe that coconut oil has been elevated as a 'superfood' without proper evidence to back it up. All fats and oils contain a mix of fatty acids, and coconut oil is no different. What may surprise you is that coconut oil is made up of about 86% saturated fat[41] — more than butter, lard or fatty meat!

DID YOU KNOW?

Replacing other fats with coconut oil goes against dietary recommendations from the British Heart Foundation[42], Heart UK[43] and the Department of Health[44]. It's perfectly fine to consume as part of your daily saturated fat intake, but don't assume it's superior to other vegan fats and oils.

Saturated fatty acids are considered unhealthy because they tend to raise the bad cholesterol in your blood, making you more at risk of heart disease, but some fatty acids have a stronger cholesterol-raising effect than others. Coconut oil evangelists assert that the type of fatty acids found in coconut oil don't have this damaging effect on our heart health.

RESEARCH

The British Nutrition Foundation reviewed the research behind many of the reported health claims around coconut oil[45] and found that there's a large amount of evidence to show that the main fatty acids found in coconut oil actually *do* increase total blood cholesterol, including 'bad' LDL cholesterol.

GETTING
YOUR FATS
STRAIGHT

CHOOSE THESE

Mono- and
poly-unsaturated fats.

Found in rapeseed
and olive oil, avocados,
nuts and nut butters.

INSTEAD OF THESE

Saturated fats
(generally solid
at room temperature).

Found in coconut oil
and palm oil.

CUT DOWN ON THESE

Fats high in
omega-6 fatty acids.

Found in sunflower,
corn, soyabean and
safflower oil.

AVOID THESE

Trans fats.

Found in some
processed foods like
cakes, pastries, biscuits
and fast food. Look for
'hydrogenated' fat or oil
on the label.

How much fat do you need?

Approximately one third of your daily calories should come from
fat, which means about 70g fat per day for women and 90g for men.
Saturated fats should only make up a third of this intake, and it's
recommended that women have no more than 20g saturated fat,
and men no more than 30g a day. Basically, cut down on saturated
fats and replace them with unsaturated fats.

SAVVY TIP

The fat in avocado is over 90% unsaturated fat.

We need fat in order to absorb fat-soluble vitamins like vitamin A and E, so I always recommend adding some good fats in the form of a dash of oil, small amounts of nuts, tahini or avocado to vegetable dishes to help absorb the maximum fat-soluble vitamins in plant foods. While animal products are the only natural source of vitamin A, the good news is that the body can actually convert the beta-carotene in plant foods into vitamin A. Sources of beta-carotene include dark-green leafy vegetables like kale and spinach, as well as bright orange vegetables like carrots, sweet potatoes, winter squash and orange and yellow peppers. The process of cooking or adding fats to these veggies improves the absorption of beta-carotene, so carrots and peppers stir-fried in oil provide more vitamin A than they would in their raw state.

THOUGHT LIFTER

You might hear that national guidelines have changed from time to time. Yesterday it was off the table and today it's all the rage. Nutrition is an evolving science – trust reputable sources and embrace evidence-based discoveries.

RESEARCH

Research published in the British Journal of Nutrition[46] in 2012 explored how adding fat to carrots affected the bioavailability of beta-carotene (i.e. the body's ability to absorb and make use of it as vitamin A). They estimated this at 11% for raw carrots compared to 75% for stir-fried carrots. The authors concluded that you could get six and a half times the amount of vitamin A from the carrots by stir-frying instead of eating them raw.

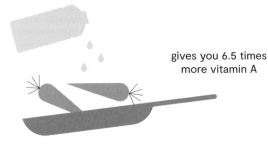

Stir-frying carrots gives you 6.5 times more vitamin A

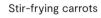

GOOD PLATE		NUTRIENT BRIDGE		SAVVY PLATE
Soup	+	Chopped nuts instead of croûtons	=	✓
Salad	+	Olive or rapeseed oil dressing and a sprinkle of chia seeds	=	✓
Sandwich	+	Smashed avocado instead of dairy-free spread	=	✓
Thai curry	+	Peanut butter to thicken	=	✓
Sweet potato mash	+	A drizzle of oil or added nuts or seeds (to help the absorption of vitamin A)	=	✓

CHOOSING 'BETTER-FOR-YOU' OILS

CHOOSE THESE

Rapeseed oil

Flaxseed oil

Hemp oil

Olive oil

Peanut oil

CUT DOWN ON THESE

Coconut oil

Palm oil

Hydrogenated oil and trans fats

Shopping for fats

PANTRY ESSENTIALS

Rapeseed oil

Olive oil

Chia seeds

Ground flaxseeds (linseeds)

Hemp seeds/ hearts

Nut butters

Nuts, especially walnuts

Soya and linseed bread

FRIDGE AND FREEZER ESSENTIALS

Frozen edamame beans

Avocado

Dark green leafy vegetables

Sesame tahini

Omega-3-fortified vegan foods

Hemp-based milk alternatives

Non-dairy spreads fortified with vitamin E or containing omega-3 fatty acids

Your fats checklist

☐ Choose foods high in unsaturated, not saturated, fats.

☐ Cook with unsaturated oils like rapeseed oil (which give you omega-3 fatty acids) instead of corn or sunflower oil (rich in omega-6 fatty acids).

☐ Olive oil has a low smoke point, so save it for drizzling onto vegetables or as a salad dressing.

☐ If a recipe includes coconut cream or canned coconut milk, opt for light varieties or replace some of the coconut with a cornflour paste or vegan instant mashed potato, both of which can be used as thickeners.

☐ Replace coconut oil with unsaturated oils, and where a recipe calls for coconut oil specifically (for taste or aroma) then use small amounts only.

☐ Check food labels and avoid foods containing hydrogenated fats (aka trans fats).

☐ Bridge the nutrient gap by finding ways to include omega-3 fatty acids in your meals (see page 66). If you don't feel able to meet your needs with food, take a daily vegan omega-3 supplement (250mg DHA and EPA).

PLANT POWER

Vegans who eat plenty of whole plant foods tend to have a better chance of getting the fat balance right – think avocados, nuts and seeds – and basing your diet on these healthier types of fats can help reduce your risk of cardiovascular disease.

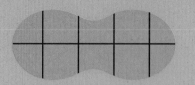

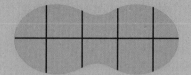

Chapter
Seven

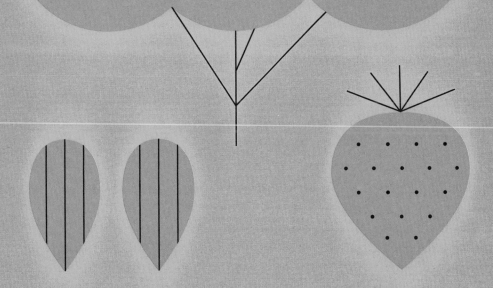

Boost Your Energy

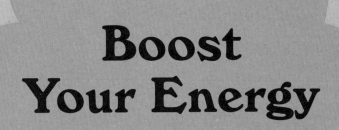

Benefits of iron

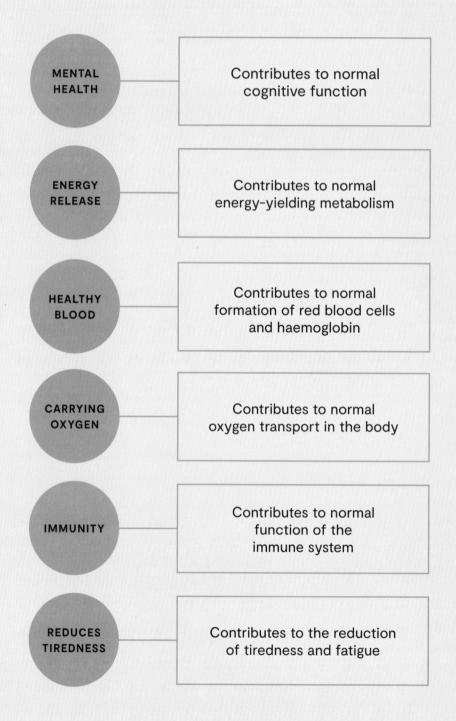

MENTAL HEALTH — Contributes to normal cognitive function

ENERGY RELEASE — Contributes to normal energy-yielding metabolism

HEALTHY BLOOD — Contributes to normal formation of red blood cells and haemoglobin

CARRYING OXYGEN — Contributes to normal oxygen transport in the body

IMMUNITY — Contributes to normal function of the immune system

REDUCES TIREDNESS — Contributes to the reduction of tiredness and fatigue

BOOST
YOUR
ENERGY

Boost Your Energy

Feeling tired? A hectic lifestyle can leave you exhausted at the end of the day, but if you find you're lethargic most of the time, it could be a sign that your diet needs attention, for example, your iron levels may be low. You don't have to eat meat to get enough iron, but you do need to think about where your iron is coming from and try to make sure that any iron you eat is being used by the body.

RESEARCH

A large study called the EPIC–Oxford study of more than 40,000 women showed that the vegans in the group did not have lower iron intakes than meat-eaters[47]. But substances such as phytates, which are found in some plant foods, can reduce the amount of iron that is available to your body.

What does iron do?[48]

Iron is needed to make the red protein called haemoglobin, found in red blood cells. Haemoglobin carries oxygen and transports it to all your cells. So, if your blood is low in iron, there's less haemoglobin, which means less oxygen for your muscles and other tissues – and this can make you feel fatigued.

How much iron do you need?

The RI of iron for adult men is 8.7mg iron/day[49] and 14.8mg for women (averaged at 14mg for food labelling). Girls and women need more because of blood loss during menstruation and those who have heavy periods are particularly at risk of iron deficiency.

Where to get plant-based iron

Foods that give you a significant source of iron will provide 15% of the RI, which means the food gives you 2.1mg per 100g (or sometimes per recommended portion). The table below lists a range of sources in descending order of the amount of iron you'll get from a typical serving.

Vegan sources of iron[51]

FOOD	PORTION SIZE	IRON (MG/PORTION)
SIGNIFICANT SOURCES		
Bran flakes, fortified	3 handfuls	5.4
Instant oat cereal, fortified	1½ handfuls	5.4
Wheat biscuits breakfast cereal	2 biscuits	4.8
Malted flake cereal, fortified	3 handfuls	4.6
Malted wheat cereal, fortified	3 handfuls	4.2
Tempeh	100g	3.6
Pumpkin seeds	2 tbsp	3.0
Baked beans in tomato sauce	1 small (200g) can	2.8
Wholewheat pasta, cooked	2 cupped handfuls	2.7
Sesame seeds	2 tbsp	2.5
Quinoa, cooked	2 cupped handfuls	2.2
Wholemeal bread	2 thick slices from a large loaf	2.1
Spinach, baby, boiled	4 heaped tbsp	2.1
OTHER USEFUL SOURCES		
Sesame tahini	1 heaped tsp	2.0
Mung dhal curry	4 tbsp	2.0
Sunflower seeds	2 tbsp	1.9
Cashew nuts	1 handful	1.9
Red kidney beans, canned	3 heaped tbsp	1.8
Lentils, cooked	3 heaped tbsp	1.7
Oats, porridge, raw	1½ handfuls	1.6
Lentil soup, canned	½ x 400g can	1.6

FOOD	PORTION SIZE	IRON (MG/PORTION)
OTHER USEFUL SOURCES		
Chickpeas, canned	3 heaped tbsp	1.5
Peas, frozen	3 heaped tbsp	1.5
Couscous, cooked	2 cupped handfuls	1.5
White pasta, cooked	2 cupped handfuls	1.4
Miso	2 tbsp	1.3
Muesli	3 handfuls	1.3
White bread	2 thick slices from a large loaf	1.3
Apricots, dried	3 apricots	1.2
Hummus	2 tbsp	1.1
Almonds	1 handful	1.1
Spring greens, boiled	4 heaped tbsp	1.1
Seaweed, nori	2 sushi sheets	1.0
Oatcakes	2 round biscuits	1.0
Hazelnuts	1 handful	1.0
Tofu	80g	1.0
Spinach, baby, raw	2 handfuls	0.9
Cooked kale	4 heaped tbsp	0.9
Dried prunes	3 prunes	0.9
Walnuts	1 handful	0.9
Chia seeds	1 tbsp	0.8
Hemp seeds	1 tbsp	0.8
Brown rice, cooked	2 cupped handfuls	0.8
Peanuts	1 handful	0.8
Raisins	1 heaped tbsp	0.7
Flaxseeds	1 tbsp	0.6
Almond butter	1 tbsp	0.6
Dark chocolate (at least 70% cocoa solids)	4 small squares	0.5
Prunes, ready-to-eat, semi-dried	3 prunes	0.4
Figs, ready-to-eat, semi-dried	2 figs	0.4
Apricots, ready-to-eat, semi-dried	3 apricots	0.4

NOTE   All beans and fortified breakfast cereals will provide some iron. Although spinach is a good source of plant-based iron, your body can only absorb small amounts, so make sure you have a bigger portion.

Making plant-based iron work for you

Iron found in plant-based foods (non-haem iron) is less well absorbed than the haem iron in animal products. So, it isn't a case of like-for-like – 10mg iron from cereal isn't as potent as 10mg iron from steak.

A compound called phytate (phytic acid) in wholegrains, some cereals, legumes, seeds and nuts binds minerals such as iron, making it less bioavailable to the body[52]. This means your body is less able to absorb and make use of the iron (see right). There's no phytate in animal products which means absorption of iron from meat is not a problem. So, you might be eating more iron than a meat-eater, but your body may actually be absorbing much less. An app that tells you you're eating enough iron according to your dietary intake therefore isn't giving you the full story!

RESEARCH

The more phytate in a plant-based meal, the less iron you will absorb. Research shows that even small amounts of phytate in a wheat roll containing 3mg iron can lead to only half the iron being absorbed[53]. The authors concluded that having vitamin C with wheat fibre would be effective in counteracting the negative effects of phytate.

You might think that the solution is to cut down on phytate by avoiding phytate-containing foods, but that would be counter-productive. One of the benefits of a plant-based diet is that it tends to be higher in fibre, and eating fewer wholegrains, legumes, and so on will reduce your fibre intake.

Taking an iron supplement as an insurance policy against compounds like phytate isn't the best solution either. Being a savvy vegan is about understanding the different interactions between plant foods and making your diet work for you by using Nutrient Bridges.

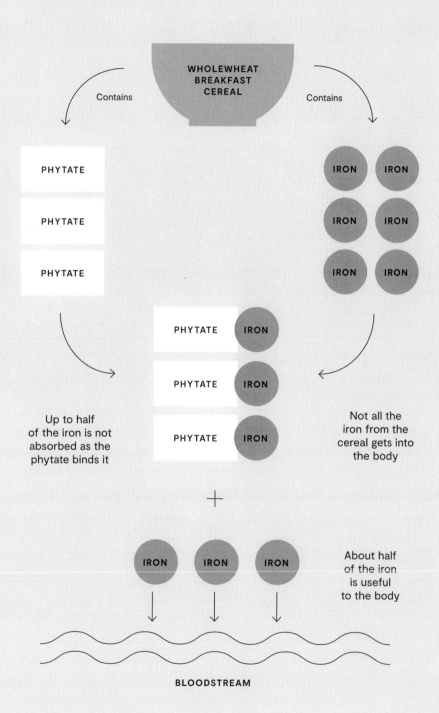

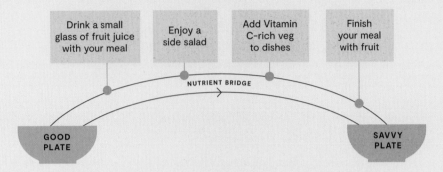

One of the biggest dietary advantages of a balanced vegan diet is the amount of fruit and vegetables you're likely to eat. They're rich in vitamin C and if you eat them alongside your plant-based iron, this markedly increases iron absorption[54]. Note – it must be at the same meal. There's little benefit to eating an orange hours before if you want to enhance iron absorption. Vitamin C works in two ways: it stops un-absorbable iron compounds from being made, and it converts iron in plant foods (ferric, or Fe^{3+}) to a more bioavailable form (ferrous, or Fe^{2+}) so it can be used by the cells[55].

PUTTING IT SIMPLY...

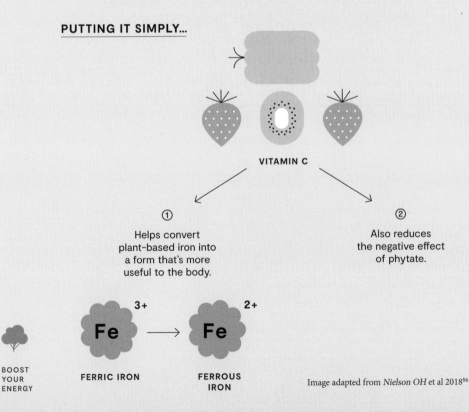

Image adapted from *Nielson OH* et al 2018[56]

Substances called oxalates in foods such as spinach are also thought to weaken iron absorption[57]. It's been suggested that we can only absorb about 1.4–7% of the iron in plants whereas we're able to absorb 20% ofthe iron in red meat[58].

ANIMAL-BASED IRON (HAEM IRON)

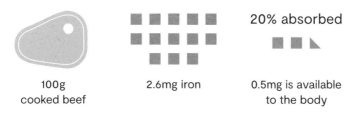

100g cooked beef	2.6mg iron	20% absorbed 0.5mg is available to the body

PLANT-BASED IRON (NON-HAEM IRON)

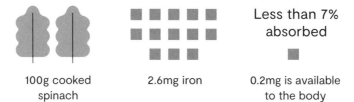

100g cooked spinach	2.6mg iron	Less than 7% absorbed 0.2mg is available to the body

---

SAVVY TIP

There are various different research findings on exactly how much iron we can absorb from plants, but the bottom line is that plant-based iron is less bio-available than haem iron.

So, even though there's the same amount of iron in both foods, if you eat the spinach your body can only make use of less than half the iron it could have used if you'd eaten the steak. This is why the vitamin C Nutrient Bridge is so important – you need to squeeze as much iron out of that spinach as possible.

Tannins in tea and polyphenols in coffee are also known to reduce iron absorption from plant foods[59]. The more tea or coffee you drink with a vegan meal, the less iron you are likely to absorb[60]. For most healthy people it doesn't seem to affect overall iron balance, but if you are at risk of low iron, then it could be worth drinking tea and coffee between meals instead. Better to drink a small glass of fruit juice to boost vitamin C (being aware that unsweetened fruit juice has around 8% sugars, so keep an eye on portion sizes). Fruit juice, whether it's freshly squeezed, chilled or UHT, has about the same amount of sugar. Freshly squeezed has a little more vitamin C but they are all great vitamin C providers, so choose whichever suits you best.

PUTTING IT SIMPLY...

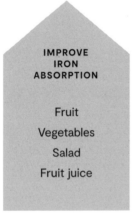

IMPROVE
IRON
ABSORPTION

Fruit

Vegetables

Salad

Fruit juice

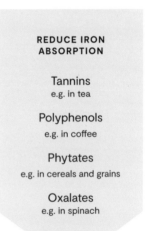

REDUCE IRON
ABSORPTION

Tannins
e.g. in tea

Polyphenols
e.g. in coffee

Phytates
e.g. in cereals and grains

Oxalates
e.g. in spinach

Dried fruits can be a good iron-provider. Semi-dried softer fruit is now more popular than traditional types. This has a higher moisture content so the amount of iron you get per 100g will be lower. Basically, if you're eating semi-dried fruit, you'll be getting less iron than if you ate 100% dried fruit.

GOOD PLATE		NUTRIENT BRIDGE		SAVVY PLATE
Iron-fortified breakfast cereal	+	150ml fruit juice, any type	=	✓
Baby spinach salad	+	Add pineapple chunks or a fresh squeeze of lime juice and increase your portion of spinach	=	✓
Stir-fried kale	+	Add orange segments	=	✓
Chickpea hummus	+	Add diced green peppers	=	✓
Mung bean curry	+	End your meal with fresh fruit (kiwi is one of the highest in vitamin C)	=	✓

And one last (slightly strange!) one... When I worked as a dietitian at Northwick Park Hospital, we had a large vegetarian South Asian population, and many of the women were low in iron. When I advised them to cook curries in a traditional cast-iron pan, their blood iron status improved! Studies in developing countries where people are iron deficient suggest that eating food cooked in iron pots can make a significant difference to the body's haemoglobin levels because tiny amounts of iron are transferred to the food[61,62].

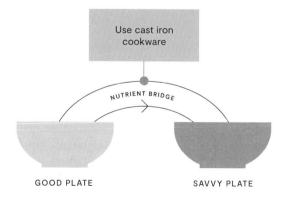

Use cast iron cookware

NUTRIENT BRIDGE

GOOD PLATE   SAVVY PLATE

This meal plan gives you a balanced day, in line with national recommendations for RIs, with lots of fibre and nearly 21mg iron to help to make up for the lower iron absorption from plant foods.

Sample menu

MEAL	FOOD	IRON (MG)
Breakfast	2 wheat biscuits	4.8
	100ml fortified soya drink	0.4
	3 dried prunes	0.9
	150ml orange juice	0.1
	1 handful of almonds	1.1
Mid-morning snack	2 tbsp hummus	1.1
	80g carrot and celery sticks	0.2
Lunch	Bean and salad wrap	3.7
	Banana	0.3
Mid-afternoon snack	2 tbsp pumpkin seeds	3.0
	1 tbsp raisins	0.7
Dinner	Vegetable, tofu and cashew stir-fry	2.4
	2 handfuls couscous	1.5
	4 small squares dark chocolate	0.5
	Total	20.7

What you get

		DAILY RI
Energy	2022Kcal	2000kcal
Fat	84g	Daily max. 70g women/90g men
of which saturates	13g	Daily max. 20g women/30g men
Carbohydrate	232g	
of which sugars	94g	Daily max. 90g
Fibre	41g	Daily target 30g
Protein	64g	Daily target 50g
Salt	3.1g	Daily max. 6g
Iron	20.7mg	Daily target 14.8mg women/8.7mg men

Three iron hacks

1.   Crush cornflakes (or other iron-fortified cereal) and use as breadcrumbs for crispy toppings to add iron to everyday foods.

2.   Drizzle lemon juice into hummus to add vitamin C; it helps you absorb the iron in the chickpeas.

3.   Build a colourful Buddha bowl salad with shredded carrots, courgette sticks, cherry tomatoes, diced green pepper, chickpeas, avocado, orange segments and a handful of almonds. The vitamin C in the fruit and vegetables will help your body make use of the iron in the almonds.

THOUGHT LIFTER

Some good news: your body is an incredible machine – when iron stores in your body are low, you start to become more efficient at absorbing it from food!

PLANT POWER

Although phytate is found in foods such as whole wheat and legumes, these foods are integral to a nutritious vegan diet. Enjoy them as part of a varied eating plan and use the Nutrient Bridges to help you become a savvy vegan – that way you have a better chance of meeting your needs for essential micronutrients.

Shopping for iron

PANTRY ESSENTIALS

Iron-fortified breakfast cereals

Dried fruit

Quinoa

Wholemeal bread

Beans and lentils

Nuts and nut butters

Seeds

FRIDGE AND FREEZER ESSENTIALS

Tempeh

Tofu

Sesame Tahini

Hummus

Spinach

Broccoli

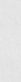
Kale

Peppers

Frozen veg

Berries

Limes and lemon

Kiwi fruit

Unsweetened fruit juice

Citrus dressing

Lemon juice

BOOST YOUR ENERGY

Energy is about more than iron...

Getting enough calories

We get energy from the calories burned when we eat macronutrients – carbs, fats and proteins. We all need different amounts of energy depending on our activity levels, genetic make-up, age, size and gender. The more active you are, the more calories you need. Public Health England recommends[63] that we distribute our daily calories throughout the day: around 400 calories for breakfast, 600 for lunch and 600 for dinner, with the rest coming from between-meal snacks and drinks.

When you stop eating meat and dairy, it's likely you'll be taking in fewer calories. Many young vegan women I see are surviving on salads, vegetable stir-fries and soups, which are nutritious but usually low in calories. They're not hungry but they often complain of being tired. Not getting enough calories can zap your energy.

It can be a challenge for some vegans to get enough calories, as plant foods tend to be bulkier and higher in fibre, so it can be physically difficult to eat enough – this can be a particular concern if you're active.

So, consider healthful ways to keep your calories to an ideal level. And if you need to increase your calorie intake, choose foods rich in healthy fats like nuts, seeds, avocado and nut butters and increase your portion size of whole plant foods like beans, lentils, vegetables and whole grains.

HOW MANY CALORIES DO YOU NEED?

An average man needs around 2500kcal a day to keep to a healthy body weight, while an average woman needs around 2000kcal[64]. UK food labels use an average of 2000kcal for the RI for adults[65]. So, if a food gives you 500kcal per portion, it's providing a quarter of your daily calorie needs.

If you're eating mainly processed and takeaway vegan foods, you may be getting plenty of calories, but these foods are often loaded with salt and not enough nutrients. Eating too much of the wrong foods can also make you feel lethargic! If you're overweight, cutting down on calories and being more physically active can help you reach a healthier weight. Research suggests that plant-based diets are a plus when it comes to preventing obesity and obesity-related conditions, as they are generally lower in calories.

HANDFUL OF PEANUTS

PIECE OF FRUIT

(e.g. orange, pear, medium banana)

MUG OF POPCORN

(try homemade with less sugar and salt)

OATCAKE SPREAD WITH YEAST EXTRACT AND HUMMUS

HANDFUL OF DRIED FRUIT

DAIRY-FREE YOGURT ALTERNATIVE

with berries and 1 tbsp of fortified breakfast cereal

BERRY AND OAT SMOOTHIE

Berry and oat smoothie made from dairy-free milk alternative, berries, 1 tbsp oats and a drizzle of maple syrup

APPLE WEDGES DIPPED IN NUT BUTTER

SNACK ATTACK BOX

Olives, broccoli florets, cherry tomatoes, carrot sticks

EDAMAME PODS WITH DIPPING SAUCE

BOOST
YOUR
ENERGY

RESEARCH

Results from research on 38,000 people participating in the EPIC-Oxford study revealed the lowest BMI was amongst the vegans in the group.[66]

What about B vitamins?

Did you know that there are eight forms of B vitamins? They are vitamin B1 (thiamine), B2 (riboflavin), B3 (niacin), B5 (pantothenic acid), B6 (pyridoxine), folate/folic acid, B12 and biotin. They have several functions, and each vitamin has its role in the body, but in essence they help convert the food you eat into fuel.

Most B vitamins

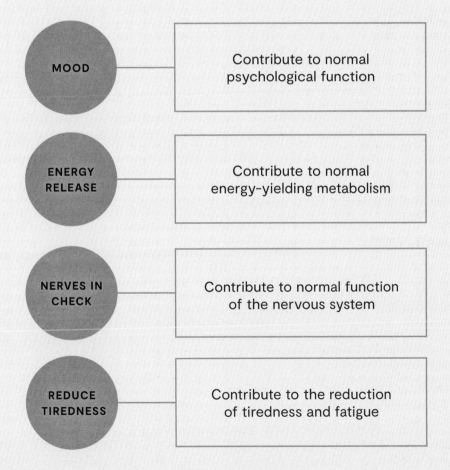

MOOD — Contribute to normal psychological function

ENERGY RELEASE — Contribute to normal energy-yielding metabolism

NERVES IN CHECK — Contribute to normal function of the nervous system

REDUCE TIREDNESS — Contribute to the reduction of tiredness and fatigue

Vegan sources of B vitamins

THIAMINE (B1)	Peas, fresh and dried fruit, wholegrain breads and fortified breakfast cereals, yeast extract, nutritional yeast flakes; white and brown flour is fortified with thiamine.
RIBOFLAVIN (B2)	Fortified breakfast cereals and brown rice, yeast extract, nutritional yeast flakes, fortified plant-based drinks.
NIACIN (B3)	Wholemeal bread and fortified breakfast cereals, yeast extract, nutritional yeast flakes. White and brown flour is fortified with niacin.
PANTOTHENIC ACID	Potatoes, oats, tomatoes, broccoli, brown rice, wholemeal bread, nutritional yeast flakes.
PYRIDOXINE (B6)	Wholegrain cereals, brown rice, peanuts, soya beans, bread, fortified breakfast cereals, nutritional yeast flakes.
FOLIC ACID	Vegetables and fruits, (including broccoli, Brussels sprouts, leafy greens, chickpeas, red kidney beans, lentils and oranges), brown rice, quinoa, fortified breakfast cereals, yeast extract, nutritional yeast flakes, some nuts (cashew, hazelnuts, walnuts) and seeds.
VITAMIN B12	Fortified breakfast cereals and fortified vegan foods, yeast extract, nutritional yeast flakes.
BIOTIN	The good news is that your gut bacteria make biotin for you from a range of foods!

Water

Sometimes feeling tired is simply due to mild dehydration. If you're feeling tired, moody or hungry, make fluid your default solution. Reach for some water, sugar-free squash, sparkling waters, dairy-free milk alternative or a vegetable smoothie. The Vegan Society Eatwell Guide[67] recommends we drink 6–8 glasses of fluid a day. You can also eat your fluids – think cucumber and watermelon!

THOUGHT LIFTER

Try drinking a glass of water every morning before you start your day and notice if you feel any different after a week.

BOOST
YOUR
ENERGY

Your energy checklist

☐ Choose iron-rich foods and combine them with foods high in vitamin C.

☐ Eat regular, varied meals and healthy snacks to keep your blood sugar levels steady and ensure a regular supply of energy throughout the day.

☐ Drink 6–8 glasses of fluid every day.

☐ Go easy on sugar-rich foods and drinks that give you a temporary energy boost – there's usually an energy slump afterwards.

☐ Avoid large, rich meals that make you feel sleepy and lethargic.

☐ Enjoy plenty and a wide range of fruit and vegetables.

☐ Choose 'better-for-you' carbs like wholegrain breads and cereals, brown rice, quinoa and brown pasta.

☐ Enjoy foods fortified with iron and B vitamins.

Lastly, feeling energised isn't just about what's on your plate.

☐ Take time out to relax.

☐ Be physically active.

☐ Get enough good-quality sleep.

☐ Explore your mental well-being.

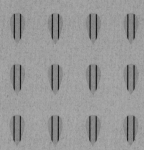

Chapter Eight

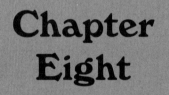

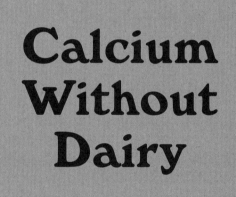

Calcium
Without
Dairy

Benefits of calcium

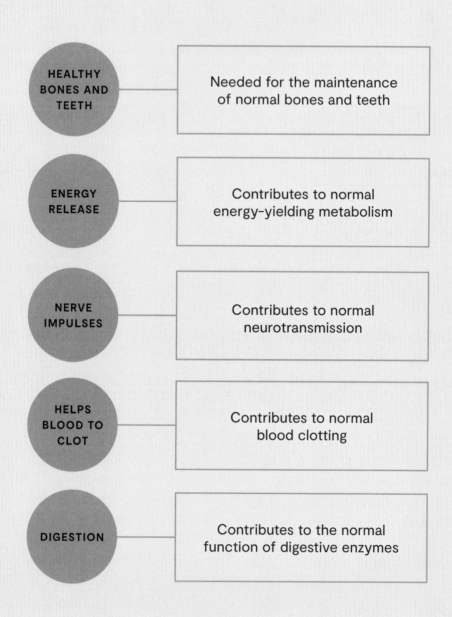

HEALTHY BONES AND TEETH — Needed for the maintenance of normal bones and teeth

ENERGY RELEASE — Contributes to normal energy-yielding metabolism

NERVE IMPULSES — Contributes to normal neurotransmission

HELPS BLOOD TO CLOT — Contributes to normal blood clotting

DIGESTION — Contributes to the normal function of digestive enzymes

CALCIUM
WITHOUT
DAIRY

Calcium Without Dairy

Why do we need calcium?

Did you know that you're probably not sitting on the same bones you were about ten years ago? Bone is constantly being broken down and built-up in a remodelling process that helps your skeleton support the structure of your whole body. Old bones are continually being replaced by new ones; this happens fastest during puberty and slows down with age.

Your diet and level of physical activity have a huge impact on the strength of your bones, and although you need a variety of different nutrients (such as vitamin D, magnesium, potassium, vitamin K and protein) to maintain bone health, around 99% of the calcium in your body is stored in your bones, making it a crucial nutrient for bone health. Calcium is also vital for helping muscles like your heart contract properly and for regulating blood clotting (the process that stops cuts and wounds from bleeding profusely).

How much calcium do you need?

Adults over nineteen years need 700mg calcium a day[68]. A diet lacking in calcium, protein and vitamin D can lead to weak bones and put you at risk of osteoporosis.

DID YOU KNOW?

Recent figures from the National Diet and Nutrition Survey suggest that teenage girls are most likely to have lower calcium intakes[69,70].

Calcium can be lost through urine, though research suggests that eating plenty of fruit and vegetables can reduce such losses. A varied diet that's rich in fruit and vegetables may offer some protection[71], but you should remain conscious of meeting your daily calcium needs.

Where to get plant-based calcium

While dairy is one of the richest sources of calcium, that doesn't mean that without it your diet will be calcium deficient. In fact, some non-dairy alternatives to milk, yogurt and cheese have been fortified with calcium to the same extent as dairy products – just don't assume you're automatically going to meet your daily needs when you make the switch and always check and compare labels to find the best option.

Organic dairy milk has been shown to be 50% higher in omega-3 fatty acids than regular (non-organic) milk, and it may also have slightly more iron and vitamin E[72]. But when it comes to plant-based milk substitutes, I haven't seen any evidence that organic versions are nutritionally superior to ones that have been fortified. We're used to assuming that when a food has something added to it, it's been adulterated and should be avoided. But when it comes to fortification of dairy alternatives, it's a definite plus if a label says 'added' vitamin B12, iodine or calcium.

DID YOU KNOW?

Terms like 'milk', 'cheese' and 'yogurt' are protected by EU law, meaning that plant-based drinks cannot be marketed as milks[73], and vegan-style 'cheese' isn't cheese at all — a helpful reminder that vegan alternatives don't always have the same nutritional qualities as their dairy counterparts.

DAIRY MILK VS. VEGAN DRINK

Calcium-fortified dairy milk alternatives typically contain the same amount of calcium as dairy milk. When there is no information on calcium content, I tend to assume that there is none added or that if there is some it is not enough to allow the brand to claim the drink is a source of calcium.

Where possible, always choose non-dairy drinks with added calcium. If you're looking for a substitute for cow's milk, you want it to provide at least a comparable amount of calcium. Some soya drinks have been fortified with tricalcium phosphate or calcium carbonate.

CALCIUM
WITHOUT
DAIRY

RESEARCH

A study published in 2000 looked at the bioavailability of calcium from drinks containing tricalcium phosphate. The authors concluded that these soya drinks, despite being fortified with calcium, are not a like-for-like comparison to dairy milk in terms of calcium absorption. They suggest that the label may be over-estimating calcium by 50%[74]. So, check the ingredients label and nutrition claims carefully.

A small study on women published in the *Journal of Nutrition* in 2005[75] suggested that the bioavailability of calcium from fortified soya drinks containing calcium carbonate is equivalent to cow's milk.

There's lots of confusion around soya, for example, regarding whether too much soya is bad for you – jump to page 42 to read more about this.

It's a little-known fact that calcium can sink to the bottom of some fortified non-dairy drinks. Some brands add stabilisers such as gellan gum to their milk-alternatives, so check the label or simply shake to be sure.

RESEARCH

It's not just about bioavailability. A US study of eight brands of fortified soya milk alternatives showed that unshaken drinks only gave you about 30% of the calcium content declared on the label. Shake the carton and they found the amount of calcium almost doubled![76] They found there was a residue of calcium left at the bottom of the carton.

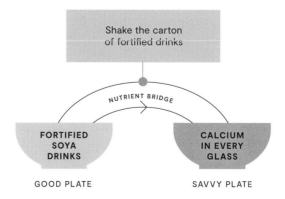

Most on-the-fence omnivores or new vegans struggle giving up cheese and, let's be honest, there's no alternative yet that beats a strong Cheddar or creamy Brie. Flavour and texture aside, many vegan cheese alternatives currently don't match up when it comes to calcium, protein, B12 and iodine levels either. All vegan products aren't created equal, so pay attention to labels when choosing your 'cheese' fix.

I've compared the labels of Cheddar with the average of three leading vegan cheese substitutes currently on the market to help you understand what to look for when making nutrient comparisons. A 30g serving is around the size of a matchbox.

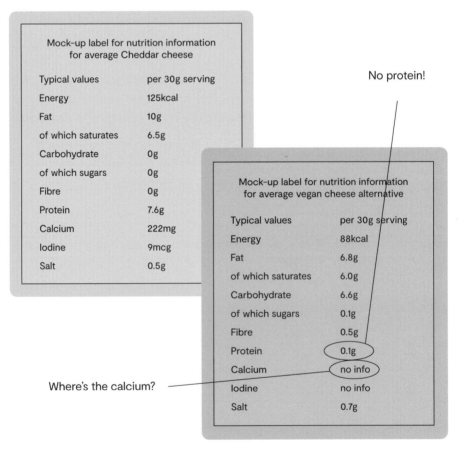

Mock-up label for nutrition information
for average Cheddar cheese

Typical values	per 30g serving
Energy	125kcal
Fat	10g
of which saturates	6.5g
Carbohydrate	0g
of which sugars	0g
Fibre	0g
Protein	7.6g
Calcium	222mg
Iodine	9mcg
Salt	0.5g

No protein!

Mock-up label for nutrition information
for average vegan cheese alternative

Typical values	per 30g serving
Energy	88kcal
Fat	6.8g
of which saturates	6.0g
Carbohydrate	6.6g
of which sugars	0.1g
Fibre	0.5g
Protein	0.1g
Calcium	no info
Iodine	no info
Salt	0.7g

Where's the calcium?

CALCIUM
WITHOUT
DAIRY

1.   When I looked at three leading brands, I found that there was no information on calcium (or iodine) content, which often implies there's none!

2.   Take a closer look and you'll find that there's next to no protein in the vegan alternatives. So, don't be misled into thinking that your plant-based 'cheese' and tomato sandwich will give you anywhere near the amount of protein as a regular version. Luckily there's about 5g protein in a thick slice of wholemeal bread, but you'll still need to supplement your meal with, for example, some nuts, seeds or beans to make sure you get a decent amount of protein compared to a regular cheese sandwich.

3.   You might assume that dairy products, being animal-based, are always going to be higher in saturated fat than plant-based versions. But this analysis shows that they're very similar. That's because many vegan alternatives are made from coconut oil, a saturated fat. We should aim to cut down on saturated fats and replace them with foods providing unsaturated fats (see pages 68–73).

REMEMBER

Don't assume vegan alternatives to dairy will meet your calcium or protein needs (or provide other dairy-associated nutrients like iodine), even if they're marketed as 'yogurt' or 'cheese'. The good news is that vegan cheese and other dairy alternatives are constantly being reformulated – and getting tastier.

THOUGHT LIFTER

It's fine to go slow, just don't stop. Make incremental changes every day and acknowledge your successes.

From the table below, you can see that, currently, fortified yogurt alternatives and soya versions declare they have almost the same amount of calcium as dairy yogurt. Unfortified versions probably have none.

YOGURTS	Dairy yogurt, low-fat, plain (150g)	Coconut yogurt alternative, fortified with calcium (150g)	Soya yogurt alternative, plain (150g)	Soya yogurt alternative, fruit, fortified (150g)	Coconut yogurt alternative, unfortified (150g)
CALCIUM (MG/ PORTION)	243	210	180	180	no info

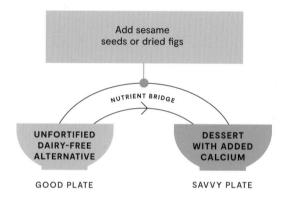

GOOD PLATE   SAVVY PLATE

Savvy shopping:
three things you must do

1. Check the packaging to see if the product says 'fortified' or if it has added calcium.

2. Look at the nutrition table and compare brands. Choose the one with the most added calcium per 100g.

3. Go beyond calcium. Compare protein, vitamin B12 and iodine too. There's a summary table of nutrient comparisons of dairy versus vegan alternatives in the Master Shopping and Nutrient Guide on pages 160–167.

Where else do you get calcium from?

This list shows you how much calcium you get from a typical serving of a particular food. The higher up the list, the greater the calcium per portion.

Vegan sources of calcium[77]

FOOD	PORTION	CALCIUM (MG/PORTION)
SIGNIFICANT SOURCES		
Instant oat cereal, fortified	1½ handfuls	601
Tofu, firm, calcium set	8g	320
Plant-based drink, fortified	200ml	240
Tofu, firm, set with nigari[78]	80g	226
Kale, boiled	4 heaped tbsp	185
Soya yogurt alternative, plain or fruit, fortified	150g	180
Sesame seeds	2 tbsp	161
White bread	2 thick slices from a large loaf	136
Sesame tahini	1 heaped tsp	129
Soya and linseed bread	1 slice	121
Tempeh	100g	120
OTHER USEFUL SOURCES		
Sesame snaps	30g	98
Wholemeal bread	2 thick slices from a large loaf	93
Baked beans in tomato sauce	1 small (200g) can	84
Almonds	1 handful	81
Figs, dried	2 figs	75
Okra, boiled	16	74
Edamame	3 heaped tbsp	70
Watercress	2 handfuls	69
Chia seeds	1 tbsp	63
Spring greens, boiled	4 heaped tbsp	60
Pak choi, steamed	4 heaped tbsp	58
Figs, ready-to-eat, semi-dried	2 figs	57
Silken tofu	80g	39
Almond butter	1 tbsp	38
Oranges	1 medium	38
Broccoli, green, steamed	2 broccoli florets	35
Sunflower seeds	2 tbsp	36

The amount of calcium in tofu varies according to the type and brand, but the figues taken from UK and US professional datasets suggest that the best types for calcium are firm tofu, set with calcium or nigari.

Loss of calcium or 'the antinutrient effect'

Research into the bioavailability of calcium (how effectively the body absorbs calcium from food) suggests that our bodies aren't able to make full use of the calcium in some plant-based foods and drinks.[79] Further, when you're not eating meat and dairy — both foods that facilitate the absorption of certain nutrients — the levels of nutrients your body actually receives can be even lower.

Phytates found in some cereals, grains and beans actually *reduce* the absorption of minerals and trace elements like calcium, iron, zinc, selenium, copper and manganese. Some people call these 'antinutrients'. But the good news is that a vegan diet is also rich in fruit and vegetables and the vitamin C from these foods can reduce the negative effect of phytates.[80] Beans and pulses are a nutritious (and cost-effective) part of a varied plant-based diet, and here's a Nutrient Bridge you can implement to minimise the effects of phytates in dried beans:

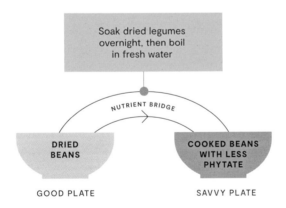

Spinach, rhubarb and Swiss chard contain another antinutrient called oxalates, a natural substance that reduces your body's ability to absorb iron and calcium.[81] According to the British Dietetic Association's One Blue Dot Reference Guide for Dietitians[82], the absorption of calcium in high-oxalate vegetables such as spinach and Swiss chard can be as low as 5%. In contrast milk, and milk products, have a bioavailability of about 30%[83], which means your body can use about six times more calcium from milk products than from spinach.

It's a common misconception that spinach is a good provider of calcium and iron. While you may think you're eating an iron- and calcium-rich food, the presence of oxalates means that your body isn't able to make full use of the calcium and iron it contains. That's not to say you should avoid leafy greens, but rather increase your portion size to ensure you get as much of the available calcium and iron as possible. Creating a smoothie from raw spinach doesn't get rid of the oxalates, so it may not be as nourishing as you might think.

Here's some good news: nutrition is an evolving science, so emerging research helps us to question previous findings. There's growing (though limited) evidence that diets high in phytate may not necessarily adversely affect nutrient intakes.[84] It's been suggested that over the long-term the body adapts to a diet rich in high-phytate foods by improving absorption rates. While studies are on vegetarians, not vegans, this adaptive effect could very well help to protect against nutrient deficiency.

DID YOU KNOW?

Women require more calcium when they're pregnant, so the body naturally increases calcium absorption at this time.[85]

Vitamin D

I can't talk about calcium without talking about vitamin D, since it's vital for your body's absorption of calcium. Without it, your body can't use much of the calcium that you're consuming. There are two types of vitamin D: D2, which is used to fortify foods, and D3, which your body produces when exposed to the ultraviolet rays from the sun and is also found in some animal foods such as oily fish.

No matter how varied your diet is, you can never get as much vitamin D from food as you can from good old sunshine, since those glorious UVB rays convert a compound in your skin (called 7-dehydrocholesterol) into vitamin D3. Remember, UVB rays are at their strongest when the sun is directly above you (when your shadow is at its shortest), so that's the best time to get out and about. This is usually around lunchtime.

Sun directly above

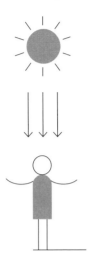

Shorter Shadow =
more vitamin D
produced

SAVVY TIP

The more skin you expose to the sun, the more vitamin D your body can produce. We do all need to protect our skin from the sun, but overdoing the sunscreen limits your body's ability to make vitamin D. It's not known how much time we need to spend in the sun to make enough vitamin D, but remember to cover up or protect your skin with sunscreen if you are sensitive or your skin starts to turn red. I recommend my patients spend 15–20 minutes in the sun every day in the summer months, especially when their shadow is shorter than them. But you're the best judge of whether this amount is too much for you.

The amount of vitamin D your body produces depends on how strong the UVB rays are, so if you live in the Northern hemisphere, where you don't get sunshine all year round, spend most of your time indoors or cover most of your body when outside, you're probably not getting enough sunshine for adequate vitamin D production. Similarly, if you're dark-skinned, you need more sunshine to make the same amount of vitamin D as someone with paler skin. Cancer Research UK[86] suggests that fair-skinned people need only a little time in the sun to make enough vitamin D in summer, but those with darker skin may need up to 25 minutes a day. They add that if you have dark skin, you're less likely to burn. Too much sun can increase the risk of skin cancer, so cover up if you begin to burn or turn red.

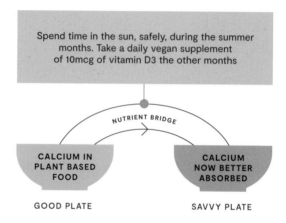

Spend time in the sun, safely, during the summer months. Take a daily vegan supplement of 10mcg of vitamin D3 the other months

NUTRIENT BRIDGE

CALCIUM IN PLANT BASED FOOD

CALCIUM NOW BETTER ABSORBED

GOOD PLATE

SAVVY PLATE

Putting it simply...

IMPROVE CALCIUM ABSORPTION

Sunshine

Vitamin D fortified foods

Vitamin D3 supplement

REDUCE CALCIUM ABSORPTION

Phytates
(e.g. some cereals, legumes)

Tannins
(e.g. tea)

Oxalates
(e.g. spinach)

Caffeine
(e.g. cola)

CALCIUM WITHOUT DAIRY

Benefits of vitamin D

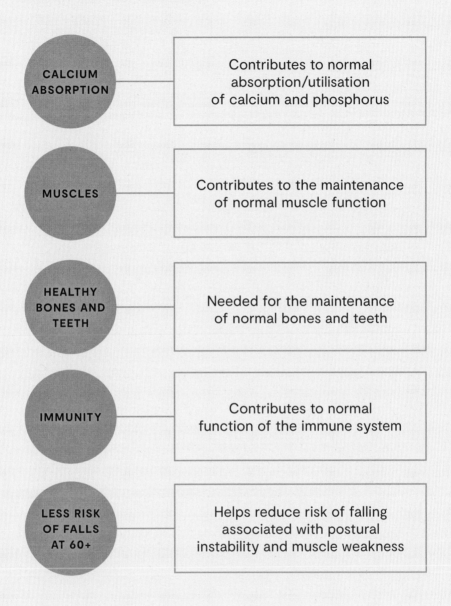

CALCIUM ABSORPTION — Contributes to normal absorption/utilisation of calcium and phosphorus

MUSCLES — Contributes to the maintenance of normal muscle function

HEALTHY BONES AND TEETH — Needed for the maintenance of normal bones and teeth

IMMUNITY — Contributes to normal function of the immune system

LESS RISK OF FALLS AT 60+ — Helps reduce risk of falling associated with postural instability and muscle weakness

Take your vitamin D supplement with your fattiest meal as it is a fat-soluble vitamin so it needs fat for better absorption. Vegan sources of fats such as avocados, nuts, nut butter and seeds are great teamed up with your vitamin D supplement.

Although phytates in foods such as wholewheat cereals and beans reduce absorption of calcium, these foods are important and nutritious components of a vegan diet and should be enjoyed as part of a varied eating plan. Vitamin C can reduce the negative effect of phytates (pages 80–81), and some studies appear to suggest your body adapts by improving absorption rates. The key is to make sure you're getting enough vitamin D so that the calcium in your diet, even from phytate-containing foods, has a better chance of being useful to the body.

Five more calcium nutrient bridges

GOOD PLATE		NUTRIENT BRIDGE		SAVVY PLATE
Yogurt alternative	+	1 handful of sliced almonds	=	✓
Jacket potato	+	Small (200g) can baked beans	=	✓
Dessert	+	Fresh orange	=	✓
Breakfast Buddha bowl	+	2 chopped dried figs	=	✓
Hummus	+	1 heaped tsp sesame tahini	=	✓

PLANT POWER

Although leafy greens, such as spinach and Swiss chard, contain oxalates that interfere with calcium absorption, remember they are still providers of other nutrients; just don't rely on them for your calcium.

This menu plan gives you more calcium than recommended to help make up for the compounds that inhibit absorption, though you wouldn't be getting this amount every day. You also get close to target amounts of fibre, saturated fat and calories.

Sample menu

MEAL	FOOD	CALCIUM (MG)
Breakfast	Porridge: 240ml fortified soya drink 40g oats 80g mixed berries	327
Mid-morning snack	150g coconut yogurt alternative	No info
	1 tbsp sunflower seeds	18
Lunch	1 tbsp ready-to-eat edamame	23
	100g mixed fruit salad	8
	Sandwich: 2 thick slices white bread 2 tbsp hummus 100g roasted vegetables	184
Mid-afternoon snack	1 handful almonds	81
	2 dried figs	75
Dinner	Rice noodles with beansprouts and pak choi	75
	Tofu, broccoli and cashew stir-fry	362
	Fresh orange	38
	Total	1191

What you get

		DAILY RI
Energy	1983kcal	2000kcal
Fat	98g	Max. 70g women/90g men
of which saturates	24g	Max. 20g women/30g men
Carbohydrate	192g	
of which sugars	68g	Max. 90g
Fibre	34g	Target 30g
Protein	67g	Target 50g
Salt	2.2g	Max. 6g
Calcium	1191mg	Target 700mg

PANTRY ESSENTIALS

Calcium-fortified instant breakfast oats

Soya and linseed bread

Seeds, especially chia, sesame and sunflower

Almonds

Dried figs

Almond butter

Baked beans

FRIDGE AND FREEZER ESSENTIALS

Calcium-fortified plant-based drinks, any flavour

Specific brands of yogurt and cheese alternatives with added calcium (check the label)

Calcium-set or nigari-set tofu and products made from tofu

Tempeh

Kale

Fresh oranges

Fresh and frozen green leafy vegetables e.g. spring greens, pak choi, watercress

Broccoli

Okra

Edamame beans

Sesame Tahini

Your calcium checklist

☐ Choose vitamin D- and calcium-fortified food and drinks, such as dairy alternatives, and have three servings of these a day.

☐ Read the fine print on labels and remember that food labelled calcium-rich should provide 30% of your daily calcium needs.

☐ Natural sources of calcium include tofu, tempeh, sesame seeds, almonds, dried figs and leafy vegetables, such as kale.

☐ Get into the habit of adding seeds and nuts to meals and try to include calcium-rich foods from the top of the *Vegan sources of calcium* table (see page 104).

☐ Experiment with calcium-set tofu and find a recipe that you can enjoy regularly. It's rich in highly absorbable calcium and good-quality digestible protein.

☐ Get out into the sunshine when your shadow is shorter than you (around lunchtime) for good vitamin D production and calcium absorption, taking care not to burn.

☐ Take a daily vegan vitamin D3 supplement (equivalent to 10mcg) in autumn and winter when the sun is not strong enough, and especially if you are dark-skinned or housebound. Have it with your fattiest meal of the day.

Bone health is about more than calcium and vitamin D

☐ Processed foods like vegan fast food or frozen vegan burgers are not off limits, but don't rely on these as a source of nutrients. They're also more likely to be high in salt, and those at risk of osteoporosis need to limit their salt intake as salt is a major factor in regulating the amount of calcium lost through urine[88]. You should have no more than 6g salt a day.

☐ Exercise regularly. Weight-bearing and resistance exercises are best for your bones, so aim for 150 minutes (2½ hours) of moderate-intensity activity a week.

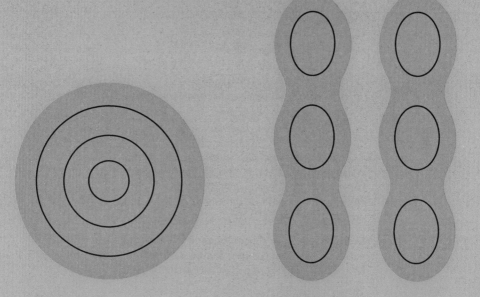

Chapter Nine

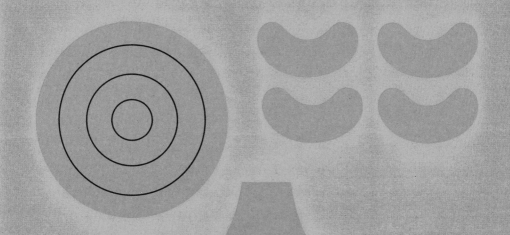

Micro-nutrients: Small but Mighty

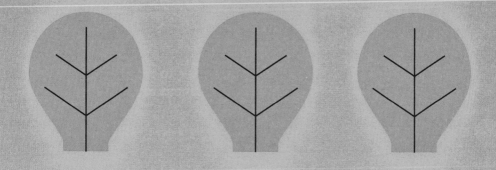

Benefits of B12[93]

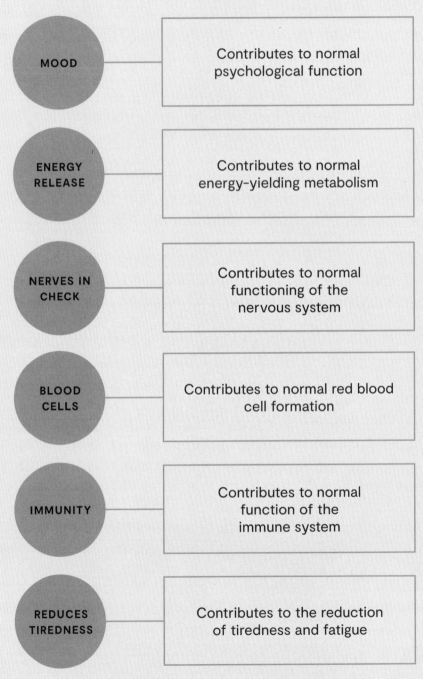

MOOD — Contributes to normal psychological function

ENERGY RELEASE — Contributes to normal energy-yielding metabolism

NERVES IN CHECK — Contributes to normal functioning of the nervous system

BLOOD CELLS — Contributes to normal red blood cell formation

IMMUNITY — Contributes to normal function of the immune system

REDUCES TIREDNESS — Contributes to the reduction of tiredness and fatigue

MICRO-NUTRIENTS

Micronutrients: Small but Mighty

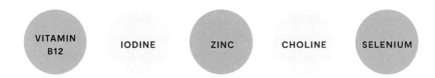

VITAMIN B12 · IODINE · ZINC · CHOLINE · SELENIUM

Eating high-quality protein, wholegrain carbs and healthier unsaturated fats is completely achievable on a well-planned vegan diet. What's often forgotten, however, is certain micronutrients that we need in small amounts, such as vitamins, minerals and trace elements. These are commonly found in animal products and some are less abundant in a plant-based diet.

You may recognise some; others are less talked about but I believe they could become more newsworthy in the future, especially if more people move towards plant-based eating and we begin to get fewer of these nutrients in the average diet. I've included them here because I think they deserve some attention in vegan diets.

Vitamin B12

Vitamin B12 is produced exclusively by microorganisms, and meat and dairy products are some of the prime sources[89]. Fortified foods and supplementation are the only vegan sources proven to be reliable.

RESEARCH

In a recent Czech study of 151 adult vegans, deficiency was prevalent amongst those who didn't take a vitamin B12 supplement. Vegans who regularly took B12 supplements had similar body levels of B12 to non-vegans[91].

HOW MUCH B12 DO YOU NEED?

The UK Reference Intake (RI) is 1.5mcg per day[92].

Vegan sources of vitamin B12[94]

FOOD	PORTION SIZE	VITAMIN B12 (MCG/PORTION)
SIGNIFICANT SOURCES		
Nutritional yeast flakes, fortified	1 tbsp	2.2
Malted flake cereal, fortified	3 handfuls (40g)	1.4
Yeast extract, fortified	1 level tsp	1.3
Instant oat cereal, fortified	1 heaped handful (45g)	0.9
Bran flakes, fortified	3 handfuls (40g)	0.9
Soya drink, fortified	200ml	0.8
Hazelnut drink, fortified	200ml	0.8
Calcium-fortified oat drink	200ml	0.8
Almond drink, fortified	200ml	0.8
Coconut drink, fortified	200ml	0.8
Rice drink, fortified	200ml	0.8
Malted wheat cereal, fortified	3 handfuls (40g)	0.8
Vegan cheese substitute (Cheddar flavour), **fortified only**	Matchbox-sized piece (30g)	0.8
Soya yogurt alternative, fortified	150g	0.6
OTHER USEFUL SOURCE		
Vegan spread, fortified	2 tsp	0.1

It's reassuring that many manufacturers of vegan products add important nutrients like vitamin B12. Be discerning when looking at nutritional information – a vegan spread may boast added B12, but you'll only get 0.1mcg in a serving and eating more isn't a healthy way to get your nutrients. However, choosing fortified spread is preferable to regular spread as it all mounts up towards your weekly B12 intake. If you want to avoid supplements, you could in theory meet your B12 needs by eating fortified nutritional yeast flakes (like Engevita) and yeast extract spreads (like Marmite and Vegemite) or other fortified products every day. You need to decide if that's practical for you.

Generally, vegans are advised to take a vitamin B12 supplement as it can be challenging to get enough from plant-based foods alone. Note that some B12 analogues may not give you the best supplementation so check the label for cyanocobalamin. The Vegan Society recommends a daily B12 (cyanocobalamin) supplement of at least 10mcg or eating fortified foods that provide 3mcg per day[95]. Recommended amounts for vegans are higher than the RI to help compensate for lower absorption rates; for better absorption, spread your B12 sources throughout the day so you're eating them in small amounts[96].

vegans are higher than the RI to help compensate for lower absorption rates; for better absorption, spread your B12 sources throughout the day so you're eating them in small amounts[96].

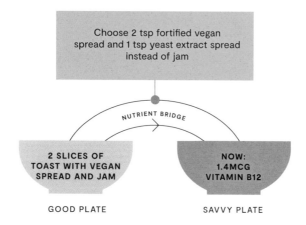

Choose 2 tsp fortified vegan spread and 1 tsp yeast extract spread instead of jam

NUTRIENT BRIDGE

2 SLICES OF TOAST WITH VEGAN SPREAD AND JAM

NOW: 1.4MCG VITAMIN B12

GOOD PLATE

SAVVY PLATE

Three nutritional yeast hacks

1. Add nutritional yeast flakes to ground cashew nuts and olive oil to make a tasty cheesy-style sauce. The BOSH! boys make a mean garlic and rosemary Camembert if you want to make your own.

2. Stir in to chilli, lasagne, soups and stews to bring umami flavours and B vitamins.

3. Sprinkle onto salads, hummus and guacamole for a nutrient boost and flavour hit.

Iodine

Milk and dairy foods are major iodine sources. The World Health Organization now classes the UK population, vegan or not, as mildly deficient in iodine[97] and the National Diet and Nutrition Survey suggests that more than a third of the iodine we eat comes from milk and dairy foods[98]. For vegans, milk alternatives that are fortified with iodine can be useful, although an analysis of thirty different brands showed that these tend to contain far less iodine than cow's milk[99].

RESEARCH

A few studies have looked at iodine intakes and body levels of iodine in vegans. A recent Norwegian study suggested that only 14% of vegans were likely to meet their iodine needs[100]. An American study of sixty-two vegans showed that urinary iodine levels were about half the iodine levels in vegetarians, indicating that vegans could be at risk of low iodine intake[101].

WHAT DOES IODINE DO?

Iodine is an essential component of the thyroid hormone thyroxine, needed for a range of bodily processes [102].Iodine deficiency can lead to reduced levels of thyroxine, which can slow down metabolism and cause weight gain, fatigue, dry skin and hair, and difficulty concentrating[103]. Even mild deficiencies in pregnancy have been associated with impaired child cognition[104].

HOW MUCH IODINE DO YOU NEED?

The UK Reference Intake (RI) for iodine is 140 mcg a day[105].

RESEARCH

The National Diet and Nutrition Survey looks at nutrient intakes of different population groups in the UK. The report published in 2018 showed that more than a quarter of teenage girls and 15% of women in the UK have very low intakes of iodine[106].

MICRO-
NUTRIENTS

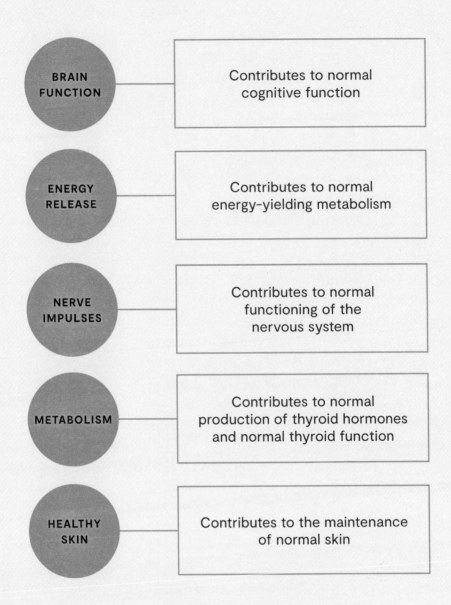

BRAIN FUNCTION — Contributes to normal cognitive function

ENERGY RELEASE — Contributes to normal energy-yielding metabolism

NERVE IMPULSES — Contributes to normal functioning of the nervous system

METABOLISM — Contributes to normal production of thyroid hormones and normal thyroid function

HEALTHY SKIN — Contributes to the maintenance of normal skin

Getting enough iodine from a vegan diet is particularly challenging, so choose fortified foods and consider a supplement. This is especially important for women planning a pregnancy as iodine is essential for development of the brain of the foetus.

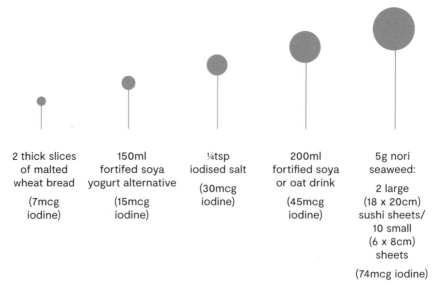

2 thick slices of malted wheat bread (7mcg iodine)

150ml fortifed soya yogurt alternative (15mcg iodine)

¼tsp iodised salt (30mcg iodine)

200ml fortified soya or oat drink (45mcg iodine)

5g nori seaweed: 2 large (18 x 20cm) sushi sheets/ 10 small (6 x 8cm) sheets (74mcg iodine)

PLANT-BASED VS. DAIRY

FOOD	PORTION SIZE	IODINE (MCG/ PORTION)
Dairy semi-skimmed milk	200ml	60
Soya drink, **fortified only**	200ml	45
Oat drink, **fortified only**	200ml	45
Soya drink, unfortified	200ml	2.0
Cheddar cheese	Matchbox-sized piece (30g)	9.0
Vegan cheese substitute (Cheddar flavour)	Matchbox-sized piece (30g)	0
Dairy yogurt, low-fat, plain	150g	51
Soya or coconut yogurt alternative	150g	0

Dairy-free drinks vary in their level of fortification, so check the label before you buy. I came across one brand of pea-based milk alternative that contained 62mcg iodine per 200ml serving, which is almost half of your daily needs, so compare brands when you're scanning shelves. I attended an insightful lecture by Sarah Bath from the University of Surrey who spoke about her research[108] into iodine-containing dairy-free drinks in the UK. She suggested choosing iodine-fortified drinks with added potassium iodide or iodate. So, look out for this on packaging.

MICRO-
NUTRIENTS

Iodised salt, which isn't currently widely available in the UK, is a good source of iodine, but too much salt is associated with greater risk of high blood pressure and strokes. Around 75% of the salt we eat in the UK comes from processed foods or food eaten away from home[109]. The daily maximum recommended salt intake is 6g a day. So, although iodised salt will give you iodine, use less than ½ teaspoon a day – and be aware that the hidden salt in supermarket and takeaway foods could be so high that you're clocking up more than 6g.

Nori roasted seaweed sheets are particularly rich in iodine and typically contain about 1.4% salt. Some brands taste very salty and in the past my advice has been to be mindful of the salt content. But, when I looked at the weight of two small (6 x 8cm) sushi roll sheets, I found they weigh just 1g and a serving gives you just 0.07g salt. So, if you were to eat ten small sheets (or two large 18 x 20cm sheets) weighing 5g, you'd meet half your daily iodine needs and get 0.35g salt. My view is that the benefit of iodine for vegans outweighs the salt issue in nori seaweed, so long as you keep within the daily salt limit of 6g (that is if you can stomach the excessive plastic some brands tend to be packed in).

WATCH OUT

The iodine content of seaweed varies, and too much iodine has been linked with thyroid problems. Do not use supplements of seaweed or kelp as an iodine source.

When it comes to iodine, it's really important not to consume more than 140mcg/day, as excess iodine can damage the thyroid gland. Brown seaweed, kombu or kelp, in particular, can be very high in iodine and the British Dietetic Association advises that seaweed, especially brown seaweed, should not be eaten more than once a week, particularly during pregnancy[110].

THOUGHT LIFTER

Choose to be grateful for all the times you've eaten well rather than guilty for the times you didn't manage it. Focus the majority of your attention on your successes.

Three nori seaweed hacks

1. Stand small nori sheets on bowls of salad or pasta to add flavour, visual appeal and crunch. No need to add salt to your meal.

2. Enjoy as an iodine-boosting snack between meals or try dipping in hummus.

3. Layer nori sheets on top of lasagne sheets when baking to add colour and flavour. Again, there's no need to add salt to your recipe.

CAN YOU GET YOUR IODINE WHEN GOING DAIRY-FREE?

At the time of writing, only fortified oat and soya drinks and fortified soya yogurt alternative can contribute to your plant-based iodine intake, and even then, the amount you'll get is less than the dairy versions. So, achieving the amount of iodine you need can be challenging on a vegan diet. The Vegan Society Eatwell Guide recommends a supplement of 140mcg iodine a day or drinking 500ml fortified plant-based drinks[111].

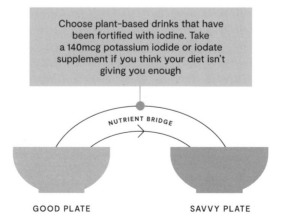

Choose plant-based drinks that have been fortified with iodine. Take a 140mcg potassium iodide or iodate supplement if you think your diet isn't giving you enough

NUTRIENT BRIDGE

GOOD PLATE

SAVVY PLATE

MICRO-NUTRIENTS

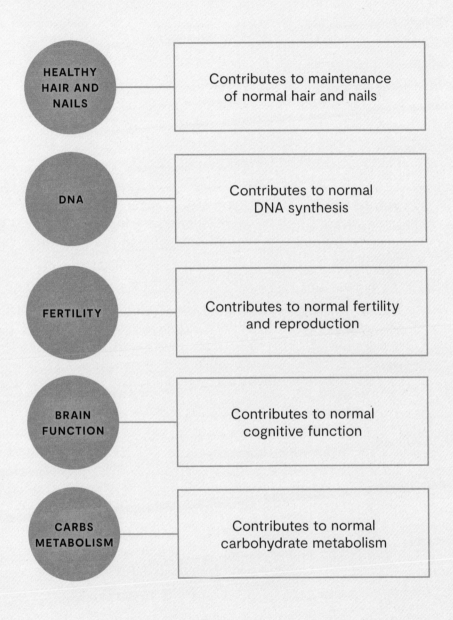

HEALTHY HAIR AND NAILS — Contributes to maintenance of normal hair and nails

DNA — Contributes to normal DNA synthesis

FERTILITY — Contributes to normal fertility and reproduction

BRAIN FUNCTION — Contributes to normal cognitive function

CARBS METABOLISM — Contributes to normal carbohydrate metabolism

Zinc

Zinc is needed for multiple processes in the body and it helps growth and development at all ages. The body doesn't have a storage mechanism for zinc, so we need a daily supply.

HOW MUCH ZINC DO YOU NEED?

The UK Reference Intake (RI) is 7mg/day for women and 9.5mg for men[113] .

WHERE TO GET PLANT-BASED ZINC

You get zinc from foods such as wheat germ (found in wholegrains), beans, nuts, seeds and mushrooms. But the amount of zinc your body can absorb (and use) varies depending on other substances in the food. Phytates can negatively affect the bioavailability of nutrients such as zinc, iron and calcium (see pages 80–81). In other words, phytates in some plant-based foods will inhibit absorption of zinc[114,115].

The EFSA advises that people who have a high intake of phytates should have corresponding higher intakes of zinc – up to 10.2mg/day for women and 12.7mg for men[116]. Foods such as black, kidney and pinto beans, nuts, seeds and wholegrains are typically some of the richest sources of phytates[117]. But don't go cutting these out of your diet – these nutritious foods form part of a healthy eating plan. The trick is to make sure you eat plenty of zinc-rich foods so that a reasonable amount is absorbed by the body. A supplement isn't necessary and could be potentially toxic if you have high doses. Simply enjoy the variety of nuts and plant-based foods that contain zinc (see the guide on pages 160–167).

Some research suggests that soaking phytate-rich foods and throwing away the soaking water can reduce the amount of phytates in them, making the nutrients more available to the body[118]. So, if you are making your own cashew cream, how about soaking the cashews beforehand?

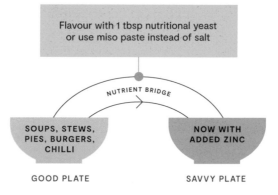

Flavour with 1 tbsp nutritional yeast or use miso paste instead of salt

NUTRIENT BRIDGE

SOUPS, STEWS, PIES, BURGERS, CHILLI

NOW WITH ADDED ZINC

GOOD PLATE

SAVVY PLATE

MICRO-
NUTRIENTS

FOOD	PORTION SIZE	ZINC (MG/PORTION)
SIGNIFICANT SOURCES		
Nutritional yeast flakes, fortified	1 tbsp	6.0
Wholewheat pasta, cooked	2 cupped handfuls	2.2
Pumpkin seeds	2 tbsp	2.0
Cashew nuts	1 handful	1.8
Tempeh	100g	1.8
Quinoa, cooked	2 cupped handfuls	1.6
Brown rice, cooked	2 cupped handfuls	1.6
Sunflower seeds	2 tbsp	1.5
OTHER USEFUL SOURCES		
Wholemeal bread	2 thick slices from a large loaf	1.4
Couscous, cooked	2 cupped handfuls	1.4
Sesame seeds	2 tbsp	1.3
Baked beans in tomato sauce	1 small (200g) can	1.2
White pasta, cooked	2 cupped handfuls	1.1
Peanuts	1 handful	1.1
Oats, porridge, raw	1½ handfuls (45g)	1.0
Hemp seeds	1 tbsp	1.0
Miso paste	2 tbsp	1.0
Spinach, baby, boiled	4 heaped tbsp	1.0
Edamame	3 heaped tbsp	0.9
Chickpeas, canned	3 heaped tbsp	0.9
Hummus	2 tbsp	0.8
Lentils, cooked	3 heaped tbsp	0.8
Walnuts	1 handful	0.8
White mushrooms, cooked	3 tbsp	0.7
Red kidney beans, canned	3 heaped tbsp	0.7
Tofu	80g	0.6
Peanut butter	1 tbsp	0.5
Chia seeds	1 tbsp	0.5
Flaxseeds	1 tbsp	0.4
Brazil nuts	3 nuts	0.4

Choline

Choline has a number of important roles. We don't hear much about choline in the nutrition press, but some researchers have called it a 'brain-building' nutrient[121].

Because choline has only recently become a nutrient of greater interest, you won't find it in professional nutrient databases or UK dietary guidelines, so it's difficult to find accurate information on which foods contain choline and how much. We also don't know enough about how much choline people are eating and also about food sources within vegan diets[122].

Eggs, meat and dairy products are good providers of choline, so plant-based diets could compromise choline intakes. We produce some choline in the liver, but this isn't enough for the body's needs, especially during pregnancy when choline requirements increase[123]. So, vegans who could be pregnant should get expert advice on monitoring their choline intake and on how to eat a varied diet that includes choline-containing foods.

HOW MUCH CHOLINE DO YOU NEED?

There are no dietary recommendations for choline in the UK, but the EFSA has set a daily adequate intake of 400mg for adults (480mg for pregnant women)[124].

WHERE TO GET PLANT-BASED CHOLINE

Researchers have suggested that pulses are a realistic source of choline for vegans[125,126]. When you look at the table opposite, based on nutrient information from sources such as the British Nutrition Foundation and NHS Digital, soya drink, soya beans, quinoa and some vegetables are the biggest choline providers. Even if you eat these daily, achieving the EFSA adequate intake of 400mg is going to be a challenge.

More research is needed on the importance of choline and whether we should be setting a daily RI, or whether certain groups should take a supplement. The good news is that the foods opposite that provide choline are also typically healthy foods that contain fibre and other nutrients. So, eating a range of nutritious plant-based foods will help you include choline in your diet.

MICRO-
NUTRIENTS

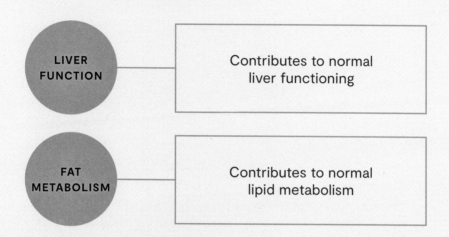

LIVER FUNCTION — Contributes to normal liver functioning

FAT METABOLISM — Contributes to normal lipid metabolism

Vegan sources of choline[127]

FOOD	PORTION	CHOLINE (MG/PORTION)
Soya drink (incl. chocolate flavour)	200ml	47
Edamame	3 heaped tbsp	45
Soya beans, roasted	1 handful	37
Quinoa, cooked	2 cupped handfuls	35
Brussels sprouts, boiled	8 sprouts	32
Broccoli, boiled	2 spears	32
Cauliflower, boiled	8 florets	31
Shiitake mushrooms	3 heaped tbsp	29
Red kidney beans, canned	3 heaped tbsp	28
Baked potato, flesh and skin	1 medium	26
Tofu, firm	80g	22
Peas, frozen, boiled	3 heaped tbsp	22
Peanuts	1 handful	19
Pumpkin seeds	2 tbsp	19
Sunflower seeds	2 tbsp	17
Mushrooms, white, cooked	3 heaped tbsp	16
Almonds	1 handful	16
Oranges, raw	1 medium	13
Peanut butter	1 tbsp	10
Almond butter	1 tbsp	8.0

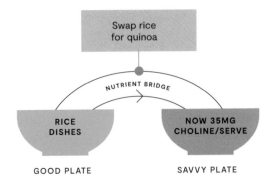

Swap rice
for quinoa

NUTRIENT BRIDGE

RICE
DISHES

NOW 35MG
CHOLINE/SERVE

GOOD PLATE

SAVVY PLATE

Selenium

Selenium has many important roles in the body.[128] Selenium isn't a nutrient of particular concern for vegans, but I've included it because, like iodine and choline, I think it is one to watch. You may remember when omega-3 was all the craze in the media – and vitamin D is one of the hot topics debated at the moment. My guess is iodine, selenium and choline may take centre stage in the future.

DID YOU KNOW?

The selenium levels in soil can vary widely depending on the type, texture and organic content of the soil which, in turn, can affect selenium levels in the foods we eat[129]. The UK used to import wheat from Canada; this wheat was rich in selenium due to the soil there. But nowadays we use more European cereals which tend to be lower in selenium[130]. Such changes mean that UK diets in general – including vegan ones – tend to be lacking in selenium.

RESEARCH

An analysis of the UK National Diet and Nutrition Survey showed that around half of women and a quarter of males aged 20–59 years had daily selenium intakes below what we call 'lower reference nutrient intakes' – the level below which deficiency could occur[131].

MICRO-
NUTRIENTS

The UK RI is 75mcg/day for men and 60mcg for women[132].

Vegan sources of selenium[133]

FOOD	PORTION	SELENIUM (MCG/PORTION)
SIGNIFICANT SOURCES		
Brazil nuts*	3 nuts	25
Chickpeas, canned	3 heaped tbsp	24
White pasta, cooked	2 cupped handfuls	20
Sunflower seeds	2 tbsp	15
Mushrooms	3 heaped tbsp	13
Brown rice, cooked	2 cupped handfuls	11
Wholewheat pasta, cooked	2 cupped handfuls	11
Cashew nuts	1 handful	8.7
OTHER USEFUL SOURCES		
Lentils, cooked	3 heaped tbsp	8.0
Soya drink	200ml	8.0
Tofu	80g	7.9
Wholemeal bread	2 thick slices from a large loaf	6.2
White bread	2 thick slices from a large loaf	6.2
Baked beans in tomato sauce	1 small (200g) can	6.0
Spinach, baby, boiled	4 heaped tbsp	5.6
Chia seeds	1 tbsp	5.5
Couscous, cooked	2 cupped handfuls	4.5
Quinoa, cooked	2 cupped handfuls	4.2

* This figure is taken from a professional database but note that Brazil nuts vary in their selenium content depending on the soil they were grown in. The Vegan Society suggests that two a day may meet your requirements[134]. Try to get your selenium from a variety of sources.

THOUGHT LIFTER

You won't be able to get everything you need in one meal. I'm a nutrition expert and even I struggle. If you include one nutrient more than you would have otherwise, you're making progress. Just do your best and don't let it stress you out.

Benefits of selenium[128]

SPERM PRODUCTION	Contributes to normal spermatogenesis
ANTIOXIDANT	Contributes to the protection of cells from oxidative stress
HEALTHY HAIR AND NAILS	Maintenance of normal hair and nails
IMMUNITY	Contributes to normal function of the immune system
THYROID FUNCTION	Contributes to normal thyroid function

MICRO-
NUTRIENTS

GOOD PLATE	NUTRIENT BRIDGE	SAVVY PLATE
Bran flakes and almond drink	Serve 40g bran flakes with 100ml (or more) B12-fortified plant-based drink. Serve with fresh berries and you'll get close to your daily **vitamin B12**.	✓
Mashed potato	Ditch the seasoning and flavour with 1 tbsp nutritional yeast and that's your daily **B12** sorted.	✓
Bowl of porridge	Make it with 200ml iodine-fortified soya drink. Add a sliced banana and you'll get nearly 50mcg **iodine**, more than a third of your daily needs.	✓
Vegan fajitas	Layer 2 large sheets (5g) of nori roasted seaweed onto the tortilla wrap before adding the filling for half your daily **iodine**.	✓
Vegetable pasta	Use wholewheat pasta and sprinkle in a handful of cashew nuts per portion – that's about half your daily **zinc** covered.	✓
Bean and lentil chilli (260g serving)	Sprinkle with 1 tbsp nutritional yeast to give you nearly 8mg **zinc**, enough for an adult woman.	✓
Handful of peanuts	Choose roasted soya nuts instead and you'll get twice the amount of **choline**.	✓
Baked potato with beans	Replace baked beans with kidney beans and serve with a glass of chocolate soya drink – that's around a quarter of your daily **choline**.	✓
Breakfast 'yogurt' and granola bowl	Add 3 chopped Brazil nuts to get ⅓ of your daily **selenium**.	✓
Vegetable rice with peas	Use brown rice, chickpeas and some sliced mushrooms. Your daily **selenium** covered.	✓

Strictly speaking you don't need to achieve all your micronutrient needs every single day; some days may be better than others. However, a daily target might make it easier to keep track. Use your common sense alongside the checklists and charts to assess how well you're doing over the week.

Your micronutrient checklist

☐ Check food and drink labels and choose those with added vitamin B12, iodine, vitamin D and calcium, especially dairy alternatives.

☐ If you don't think you're achieving 1.5mcg vitamin B12 and 140mcg iodine through fortified foods, take a supplement.

☐ Add a zinc booster to your meals with wholewheat pasta, quinoa and brown rice.

☐ Eat a wide variety of nutritious plant-based foods to help meet your choline needs.

☐ Choose foods such as chickpeas, Brazil nuts and pasta for selenium. But be aware that too much selenium can be harmful.

☐ Choose iron-rich foods and combine them with Nutrient Bridges such as foods high in vitamin C (see page 85).

☐ Take 10mcg/400i.u. vitamin D3 daily (with your fattiest meal) in the autumn and winter, and all year round if you are housebound. Expose your skin to the sun safely during spring and summer (see page 106).

MICRO-
NUTRIENTS

PLANT POWER

A vegan diet can be a savvy vegan diet by eating a good range of whole plant foods and enriching them with Nutrient Bridges.

GET VALUE FOR YOUR CALORIES

You might be taking in an appropriate number of calories for your daily energy needs, but those calories could be made up of fast food, vegan chocolate and crisps. Such foods are unlikely to give you the range of nutrients you need for good health. So, as well as considering the number of calories, it's important to think about where the calories come from. Ideally, you want to have calories with added value – vitamins, minerals, fibre, and so on.

THOUGHT LIFTER

You've haven't failed if you need to take supplements. Supplements aren't the enemy, and if it's a choice between taking a supplement or getting less than the recommended amount of a nutrient, go for the suggested dose of a supplement.

Chapter Ten

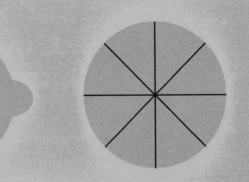

Eating In:
Building
Healthy
Habits at
Home

Eating In:
Building Healthy
Habits at Home

The beauty of plant-based eating is the potential to eat plenty of whole foods high in fibre and essential nutrients. Often that means more home cooking and fewer takeaways and pre-prepared shortcuts. But it's not always possible to cook from scratch, and sometimes you need to rely on convenient products that save time and energy; my aim is to help you get balance most of the time.

How to choose the healthier option

Some retailers and manufacturers use traffic light colour-coded labelling, which can make it quicker for you to compare foods. It's pretty self-explanatory: try to choose foods with more greens or ambers and, just like when you're driving, avoid too many red lights. Traffic lights do have limitations, for example, nuts would have a red traffic light for fat yet they certainly deserve to be in your shopping trolley.

Also look at whether any nutrients have been highlighted on the pack. A nutrient claim, such as 'source of iron' means that 100g or a recommended serving of the food will contribute 15% of your daily iron needs. If the label says 'rich source' or 'high in iron', you'll be getting 30% of your daily target. The same applies to claims about any vitamins or minerals.

You might be put off by foods that have a list of ingredients full of chemical names you don't understand. Ingredients are listed in descending order according to how much of that ingredient is present. This is really helpful when you want to know if, for example, beetroot is the main ingredient in your beetroot burger! Compare brands. Look at the labels on a couple of brands you like and choose the one that gives you less salt, sugar and saturated fat.

When I'm rushing around in a supermarket trying to find things, I'm often frustrated by 'choice overload'. Although I automatically hone in on nutrition facts, they aren't always easy to decipher. Foods don't all come in handy 100g portions, but when you look at the nutrition on a food label, the information on calories and nutrients is presented per 100g. 'Per 100g' figures are useful when you're comparing brands. 'Per portion' values will help you work out how much of those nutrients you'll actually get when you enjoy your meal.

Some manufacturers list the nutrition information per portion, and some go even further by telling you the nutritional value of a food as it is eaten, like '40g breakfast cereal with 125ml semi-skimmed milk'. This is the most useful way to help you understand what you're actually eating in that meal (as long as you eat the recommended portion size).

The portion stated isn't always the portion eaten

When a manufacturer declares the amount of nutrients and energy per portion, think about whether that matches your portion size. You may notice that you can easily munch through a whole ready meal, yet the recommended amount might be just half a pack. In which case, you need to double the nutrition information on the label to know what's in your portion.

The intel on vegan convenience foods: 'Vegan' doesn't always mean healthy

Some people mistakenly think a 'vegan' label on a food product means it's healthy. But many ready meals can be high in salt and some don't give you enough protein. Remember the VVPC plate (see page 19) and add side salads, extra vegetables or protein sources (such as beans, peas or sweetcorn) to meals that you think aren't going to cover all your nutritional needs. These accompaniments will also give you extra fibre and essential nutrients.

I scanned supermarket shelves and online data to compare over 100 different vegan products and have categorised them into groups. It's not easy to say whether they're nutritious because there really isn't much nutrition information out there on micronutrients like iodine and vitamin B12. But I've listed some pros and cons based on the data I was able to find.

FOOD*	WHAT'S GOOD	WHAT'S NOT SO GOOD
Meat substitutes in general	Some brands have added iron and vitamin B12. Products that had the highest amount of protein were based on seitan or wheat gluten.	Levels of fat, saturates, protein and salt vary a lot between brands. Choose those lower in saturates and salt.
Vegan mince (from 7 samples)	Most types are low in fat. Mince based on soya, wheat or pea protein can give you up to 20g protein per 100g. Provides fibre.	Higher in salt compared with minced meat. Mushroom-based mince has less protein than the others.
Meat-free pieces (from 6 samples)	Most are low in fat, but best to check the label. A 100g portion of most brands provides up to 20g protein. Contains fibre.	Higher in salt compared to conventional meat. So, when cooking, try not to add salt to your recipe.
Coated meat-free pieces (from 8 samples)	Many are lower in fat and saturates, protein and salt, and higher in fibre compared with chicken goujons and nuggets.	A few are high in fat or salt.
Sausages and burgers (from 39 samples)	Sausages and burgers made from mycoprotein (sold as *Quorn™*), wheat, soya or pea protein can give you about 15g protein per portion as well as providing fibre. Many (but not all) are lower in fat and saturated fats compared with conventional products.	Sausages and burgers made from vegetables or mushrooms are lower in protein, so check the labels and look for protein sources such as beans and lentils. Products that contain coconut oil can be as high in saturated fat as regular meat-based sausages and burgers. They tend to be quite high in salt.
Meat-free balls (from 5 samples)	Meat-free balls made from pea or soya protein can provide 10g or more protein per serving. Most also give you fibre. Look for pea or soya protein on the label.	Balls and bites that are made with vegetables like butternut squash, carrot and sweetcorn are lower in protein and fibre.
Sausage rolls (from 5 samples)	Those based on Quorn™ or soya have similar amounts of protein to meat-based sausage rolls. Tend to be lower in fat than conventional sausage rolls.	Some are high in salt. All are high in saturated fat. Some contain palm oil.

Meat-free 'bacon' (from 6 samples)	Choose products that are based on seitan, wheat gluten or soya as these have comparable levels of protein to conventional bacon. Some brands have added iron and vitamin B12. Contains fibre.	Most products are high in salt, as is regular bacon. Bacon made with coconut can be higher in saturated fat.
Coated fish-free pieces (from 7 samples)	Most are comparable with fish fingers in terms of fat and protein content. All give you more fibre than fish fingers.	A few products are high in fat and several are high in salt, so make sure you check the label. They are meant as fish substitutes, but don't provide the iodine you get from fish.
Plant-based tuna (2 samples)	Can be a useful source of protein. Made from peas, soya, lentils and/or chickpeas. Contain fibre.	Not widely available.
Savoury crisp-like snacks made from lentils or chickpeas (from 7 samples)	Many are higher in protein and lower in fat compared with potato crisps.	Still high in salt and some contain more salt than potato crisps, so it is important to check the label. (Regular crisps have about 1.5g salt/100g.)
Protein powder (from 10 samples)	My samples ranged from 49–90g protein per 100g powder. Generally, a serving will give you about 20g protein. Some powders are fortified and so can help to top up levels of micronutrients like vitamin B12 and iron as well as omega-3 fatty acids.	Protein content varies according to the source. Powders based on peas and beans are typically higher in protein compared with those based on hemp. Protein powders are not necessary for vegans eating a varied diet. The VVPC plate helps ensure you get protein in every meal.

* (average from a range of product samples)

**Note this comparison is based on data found at the time of writing and represents an average of various product nutrition information.

THOUGHT LIFTER

If you keep good food in your house, you're more likely to end up putting good food in your mouth. Stock the fridge and cupboards full of tasty, healthy foods. Suddenly you'll find yourself choosing between two healthy options, it's a win-win.

Protein swaps that might surprise you

Many vegan foods make great swaps for meat-based foods and some even bring rich umami flavours, but this isn't always the case. Lots of young people I work with make like-for-like switches and assume the vegan versions will provide the same nutrition. Here are six examples to help you become more nutrition savvy.

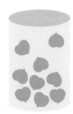

AQUAFABA INSTEAD OF EGG WHITE?

Vegan recipes often suggest aquafaba (chickpea liquid from a can) in place of egg white. Although this is a great culinary use, I don't see it as a good swap nutritionally. The protein digestibility-corrected amino acid score (PDCAAS) compares a protein's amino acid quality as well as our ability to digest it[135]. Egg protein has a high PDCAAS because it contains all nine essential amino acids and is easily digestible, making it an excellent protein source. Aquafaba has less than a fifth of the protein you'd get from egg white. So, by all means cook with aquafaba, but also include a protein source such as soya mince, beans or nuts in your meal.

CHIA-STYLE EGG OR BOILED EGG?

Chia seed egg alternative is often used in recipes to create an egg-like consistency. A tablespoon of chia seeds soaked in 3 tablespoons of water for 10 minutes can form a glutinous gel that's useful in baking. Flaxseed prepared in the same way can also make a good egg replacement in cakes and cookies, but more than a tablespoon can create a bitter aftertaste. They both provide almost a quarter of the protein you'd get from an egg.

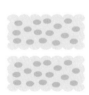

JACKFRUIT OR TEMPEH INSTEAD OF CHICKEN?

I love the fact that young green jackfruit has a similar texture to chicken and comes conveniently in a can. Look a little closer, however, and you'll find that jackfruit is virtually devoid of protein. So, whenever you're using it as a meat substitute, think about where else your protein will come from.

The good news is that three segments of canned green jackfruit count as one of your five-a-day fruit and veg and are a source of fibre. So, enjoy jackfruit as a nutritious food, but don't use it as your protein source.

Tempeh is a different matter. You get around two-thirds of the protein when compared to grilled chicken breast, so it is a good substitute.

MUSHROOMS INSTEAD OF BEEF?

Mushrooms, especially field varieties, bring a savoury umami flavour, adding rich colour and depth to dishes. I remember devouring a mushroom moussaka in Crete and not missing the meat one bit. But how do mushrooms stack up as a meat substitute? Sadly, not very well. Mushrooms won't give you the iron and B12 you get from beef, or the protein, so if you're cooking with mushrooms instead, add some nuts, tofu, Quorn™, beans, peas or lentils for your protein.

SCRAMBLED TOFU INSTEAD OF SCRAMBLED EGG?

Tofu is a good-quality, easily digested and rich source of protein, which you can use in place of animal-based proteins while still getting your goodness. Although a little lower in protein than eggs, a portion of scrambled tofu is a healthy way to start the day. Accompany with some wholegrain bread, grilled tomatoes and mushrooms, sliced avocado and a generous portion of wilted baby spinach. Delicious!

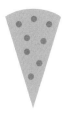

VEGAN CHEDDAR-STYLE INSTEAD OF CHEDDAR CHEESE?

I eagerly await a manufacturer that significantly improves the nutritional composition of vegan cheese alternatives. Cheese is a rich source of protein but dairy-free substitutes available today are disappointingly virtually devoid of the protein, calcium and iodine found in regular cheese (see page 100 for more nutritional comparison). Enjoy cheese alternatives but look for these nutrients in other foods instead (see chapters 4, 8 and 9).

Check the label as some brands of vegan cheese alternative have added vitamin B12 and calcium and these are better than unfortified types. Contrary to what you might think, added vitamins and minerals that make an ingredients list look more complicated are actually nutritionally beneficial. So, actively look out for meat and dairy alternatives that have been fortified.

Swap facts – the numbers

FOOD	PROTEIN (G/100G)
Aquafaba	2.4
Egg white	13.0
Chia seed mix	3.0
Flaxseed mix	3.3
Boiled egg	14.1
Jackfruit	0.5
Tempeh	20.7
Chicken	32.0
Mushrooms	1.4
Beef mince	24.7
Scrambled tofu	8.1
Scrambled egg	11.0
Vegan cheese substitute	0.4
Cheddar cheese	25.0

THOUGHT LIFTER

Surround yourself with people who are going to support you on this journey. It's harder to be a savvy vegan if you don't have anyone around you who relates to your goals and beliefs (whatever they are). Seek out people whose dietary choices inspire you.

PLANT POWER

Vegan home cooking can be super-nutritious – just spend a little time comparing food labels and make up for shortfalls in vegetables or protein.

Three leftover makeovers to bridge nutrient gaps

1. Iodine-rich Risotto: Add fortified oat drink, colourful vegetables and roasted seaweed strips to leftover boiled rice and cook thoroughly until softened and moist.

2. Omega-3 Pitta Pockets: Stuff leftovers into pitta bread with salad dressed in lime and rapeseed oil. Finish with a scattering of chia seeds.

3. B12 Quick Quesadilla: Pan-fry one side of a wholemeal tortilla wrap, turn it over, pile on your leftovers, and sprinkle with B12 nutritional yeast flakes. Place another tortilla wrap on top, smother with grated B12-fortified vegan cheese and grill.

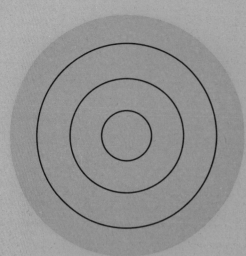

Chapter Eleven

Eating Out:

Staying Powerful When Out and About

Eating Out: Staying Powerful When Out and About

It's not always possible (or fun) to cook every meal, so this is your guide to making healthier choices when out and about.

I was recently asked to survey popular high-street lunches for a national newspaper. Most didn't match up to a healthy option in terms of calories, good fats, salt, fibre and protein for both vegan and non-vegan options. It demonstrated just how difficult it can be for you to get balance during a working day.

Grabbing lunch

You may rush to the supermarket or coffee shop, pick up a drink and a sandwich and think 'that's lunch sorted'. But a little careful thought could keep you more satisfied and energised for the rest of your busy day. Keep the VVPC plate in mind (see page 19) – it can really help you eat better when you're away from home. You may not always be able to fill all sections with something off a shelf, so check out the Savvy Sides section overleaf to supplement your meal.

GOING FOR BAKED POTATO FOR YOUR CARBS?

Enjoy a generous topping of baked beans or mixed bean and vegetable chilli to tick off your protein. Add a mixed salad or vegan coleslaw and finish with fresh fruit. VVPC sorted. The vitamin C Nutrient Bridge in the salad and fruit will help release the iron from the beans. Your good plate just got savvy!

EATING
OUT

Three top
sandwich tips

1. Go for wholemeal, wholegrain, granary, or soft grain white bread. Wholemeal wraps and pitta bread are also great choices.

2. Choose a filling that gives you protein, such as peanut butter, hummus, falafel, sweetcorn, beans, lentil pâté or meat substitutes made from soya or seitan (wheat protein).

3. Have some salad or vegetables too, either as part of the filling or on the side.

Three top salad tips

1. Make sure you have some wholegrain carbs, such as quinoa, brown rice, buckwheat, bulgur wheat, wholewheat couscous, oats, spelt or brown pasta.

2. Vegan fats can be great fats – choose avocado, nuts, nut butters and seeds.

3. Go colour mad. The more natural colours in your bowl, the wider the range of nutrients.

10 savvy sides to bridge the nutrient gap

Add these accompaniments to your meal to fill all sections of the VVPC plate.

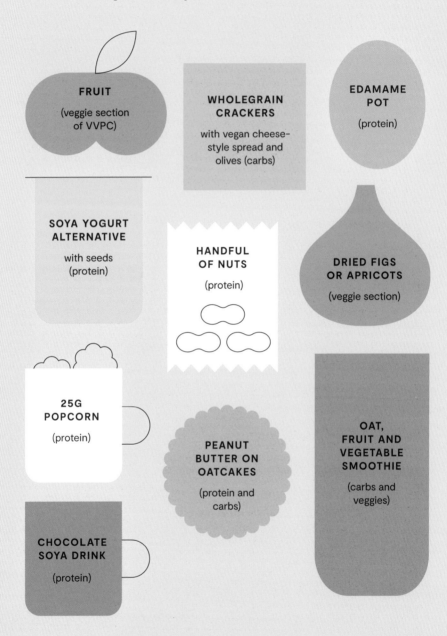

FRUIT

(veggie section of VVPC)

WHOLEGRAIN CRACKERS

with vegan cheese-style spread and olives (carbs)

EDAMAME POT

(protein)

SOYA YOGURT ALTERNATIVE

with seeds (protein)

HANDFUL OF NUTS

(protein)

DRIED FIGS OR APRICOTS

(veggie section)

25G POPCORN

(protein)

PEANUT BUTTER ON OATCAKES

(protein and carbs)

OAT, FRUIT AND VEGETABLE SMOOTHIE

(carbs and veggies)

CHOCOLATE SOYA DRINK

(protein)

THE GOOD NEWS

Many vegan options are higher in fibre than non-vegan alternatives and contribute towards your five-a-day of fruit and vegetables.

If you dine out as a treat once a week, let yourself off the hook and don't worry about the VVPC plate. Enjoy your evening out, savour the flavours, and don't feel guilty if everything on your plate is fried. We all enjoy an indulgence from time to time.

However, if you are regularly eating out, say three times a week or more, you need to be thinking about the VVPC plate. Order extra vegetables or a salad on the side or choose deep-fried foods less often. Sometimes that's not so easy, especially when vegan choices tend to be just as expensive (I've never understood why).

Fortunately, restaurants are becoming creative with their menus and there's far more choice than ever. Some have added a touch of elegance by creating culinary masterpieces from ordinary vegetables served in ways that explode with colour and ooze temptation. They also taste divine. Sharing platters can be a treasure chest of discovery. Sadly, I haven't yet seen such beautiful plates of plant-based food presented in a vegan savvy way, giving as much care to the nutritional benefits as the taste. And I strongly believe that's very possible to do.

Hold your head up high and order delicious choices with confidence; being a savvy vegan is about balance. Secondly, avoid going to a restaurant ravenous. Grab a piece of fruit or a handful of nuts before you set off. It can help stop you over-ordering unhealthy dishes. Get into the habit of putting your knife and fork down after every mouthful; eating mindfully helps you to explore the textures in a more conscious way and you might be surprised at how much more flavoursome your meal becomes. Lastly, remember you're there to enjoy yourself. So long as this isn't something you do five days a week, experiment with the range of vegan dishes on offer.

THOUGHT LIFTER

We've all heard we should treat our body like a temple, but sometimes it would rather be a nightclub, and that's OK! A little of what you fancy does you good, so embrace it. Just be mindful that too much can have consequences.

I assessed the nutrition information from thirty vegan and non-vegan meals you can order in eight leading outlets.

ENJOY COLOURFUL FILLING SALADS
Look for grains, beans and pulses, including falafels, to give you fibre and protein.

SWEET POTATOES
These are a great choice as they give you fibre and vitamin A. Choose baked ones rather than fries, which are often just as high in fat and salt as regular fries.

INDIAN
There is usually a range of vegan options available; dhal or chickpea-based curries provide protein and micronutrients. Vegetable-based curries (such as cauliflower and spinach) are lower in protein but still provide a range of minerals and vitamins.

GOING MEXICAN
A feast for the eyes, senses and palate, Mexican food can be a great move. Choose wraps, burritos and fajitas brimming with colourful vegetables like mixed peppers and onions. Say yes to refried beans. Enjoy crispy salad and guacamole on the side.

ASIAN FOOD
Chinese, Thai and Japanese dishes based on tofu and tempeh are great options, providing protein and minerals. Limit deep-fried dishes.

THE PUB MEAL
A vegetable-based curry or bean chilli provides protein, fibre and minerals. Go easy on the poppadums and tortilla chips as they can be high in salt.

BURGER 'N CHIPS
Depending on the main ingredient, a vegan burger and chips may be lower in saturated fats and higher in fibre than non-vegan alternatives. Choosing sweet and sour, barbecue or tomato sauce gives you less fat than the mayo or soured cream that's often in a regular burger.

ALL-DAY BREAKFAST
Avocado for good fats, spinach for potassium, vegetable sausages for a bit of protein (scrambled tofu is even better), a large serving of baked beans for iron, tomatoes for antioxidants and toasted sourdough or wholemeal bread on the side. Enjoy with a small glass of fruit juice in place of tea so you make better use of the iron in the spinach.

LEBANESE? YES, PLEASE
From starters to mains, grilled vegetables smothered in Middle Eastern spices are nutritious vegan options. Roasted aubergine will give you fibre, green peppers bring vitamin C and chargrilled tomatoes and onions count towards your five-a-day. Enjoy hummus and falafel for protein, plenty of mixed salads doused in zingy dressings and pitta bread for a balanced meal.

Top tips on eating out: what to look out for

1. It can be challenging to get sufficient levels of some minerals and vitamins, such as iron and zinc, so look for dishes that contain grains, nuts, seeds, beans and pulses.

2. Many vegan items may be lower in protein especially if they're mainly made up of vegetables. Order meals with good sources of protein, such as tofu, beans and meat substitutes.

3. Look out for salt. Like meat-based options, many restaurant plant-based meals can be highly salted.

4. When choosing vegan pizza or macaroni cheese, remember that vegan cheese substitutes are usually coconut-based and so probably high in saturated fats; they will also probably be lacking in minerals such as calcium and iodine. These dishes can be high in salt too.

What's so bad about salt?

Many foods eaten outside the home tend to be high in salt. Salt is made up of two parts: sodium and chlorine, combined in a compound called sodium chloride. It's the sodium which can be harmful because although your body needs a certain amount to regulate fluid in your body, too much can increase your risk of developing high blood pressure and strokes.

Whether you're reaching for table salt, pink Himalayan salt, sea salt or Kosher salt, they're all mainly sodium chloride. There is no robust evidence to suggest that one type of salt is better for you than another. Health claims about any of these trendy salts have no scientific basis and are not approved by the EFSA.

Beyond the Book: Bringing it All Together

This is your quick and easy treasure chest of tricks to maintain healthier plant-based eating long term.

The big five

Firstly, if you don't remember anything else, try to follow these top five tips:

1. Choose whole plant foods such as beans, lentils, wholegrains, fruit, vegetables, nuts and seeds in preference to fast foods and ready meals.
2. Follow the VVPC plate for main meals (see page 19).
3. Add Nutrient Bridges to your meals (see the summary of bridges on pages 158–159) – they also help you absorb nutrients from plant-based foods (below).
4. Have a portion of calcium at every meal, such as calcium-fortified dairy alternatives, tofu, tempeh, baked beans, soya beans or kale.
5. Take a vitamin D supplement as well as suggested doses of any other nutrients you're struggling to get from food (that is, if you can't manage all the Nutrient Bridges).

7 ways to increase nutrient absorption

① Eat larger portions of spinach or Swiss chard, as they have oxalates that reduce calcium absorption.

② Add vitamin C-rich foods like fruit and veg to reduce effect of phytates in wholegrain cereals and legumes – they help absorb iron and zinc.

③ Add nuts or a little oily dressing to help absorb vitamin A from raw veg.

④ Add citrus fruit, berries, peppers, tomatoes and green leafy veg to meals to increase iron absorption.

⑤ Stir-fry carrots and peppers rather than having them raw to help absorb vitamin A.

⑥ Avoid drinking tea with meals as it reduces iron absorption.

⑦ Take a vitamin D supplement with your fattiest meal of the day, as it is a fat-soluble vitamin.

Being vegan savvy just got easier. On page 160 you'll see a Master Shopping and Nutrient Guide that brings everything together:

1. Staple healthy items for your shopping trolley, categorised into 'VVPC foods'.
2. Handy tick boxes so you know which foods give you which nutrients; fibre, omega-3s, B12, iodine, they're all there at the flick of a page.

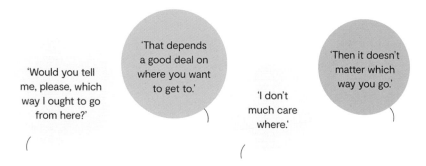

'Would you tell me, please, which way I ought to go from here?'

'That depends a good deal on where you want to get to.'

'I don't much care where.'

'Then it doesn't matter which way you go.'

You may recognise this quote from *Alice in Wonderland*. If you want to be a savvy vegan, then getting clarity on where you want to get to and why will help you to reach your goal.

To make it easier for you to eat well, the guide is categorised into 'VVPC foods'. They're also listed more or less in the order of the layout of your supermarket. Enjoy a wide variety of foods you like – this is not an exhaustive list; I've just singled out those that are nutritious and provide Nutrient Bridges. All foods will be sources of a different range of nutrients, so having a good mix will give you a better chance of having a balanced week. The foods in the VV column typically provide fibre and some vitamins and minerals. You'll notice there are lots more foods under V, as half your plate needs to be filled with these colourful fruit and vegetables. Feel free to throw any fruit or vegetables you like into your supermarket trolley; fresh, frozen, dried or canned.

Protein foods (P) are a must for every meal. The key is to have a mix across the day so you're getting all the essential amino acids, which are the building blocks of protein. Most of the carbs (C) in the list also give you fibre, and many of them bring whole grains.

Now, it's the Nutrient Bridge that makes you an especially savvy vegan. Look at the micronutrients columns in the shopping guide. They may not normally be front of mind when you're buying groceries, yet they can make the difference between a good plate and a savvy plate. If a food has two ticks, it's a significant source of that nutrient. This isn't about just the maximum number of ticks, it's about getting ticks in every column so you're buying foods with different nutrients. If a food has only two ticks overall, you might not think that's enough when you compare it to other options, but if one of the ticks happens to be selenium, it deserves a place on your list because fewer foods give you selenium. Variety is key.

Supplements are meant to *supplement* not replace

I believe the best way to get all the nourishment food has to offer is to eat real food, not to take a pill. It may be difficult for some vegans to achieve adequate amounts of certain key nutrients from their meals, so supplementation can help to safeguard against deficiency. So, I do recommend certain supplements at times if you're struggling to meet your needs. Check with a dietitian or your doctor if unsure or if you have underlying health conditions that concern you.

Unless you live in a country that's sunny all year round, a vitamin D supplement is essential in autumn and winter, no exceptions. This is especially important if you have dark skin or are housebound. Food sources of this vitamin are incredibly limited, even if they are fortified.

For the other nutrients, here are six groups of foods you must have on your shopping list if you want to try to avoid supplements. You may still need to take extra iodine, vitamin B12 and omega-3 if you're not getting enough every day from your diet, but it is possible to meet your needs if you eat the following foods regularly:

1. Citrus fruit, fruit juice (limit your free sugars to 30g a day, page 58), vegetables such as peppers and cabbage, and salad all contain vitamin C, helping you absorb iron.
2. Nutritional yeast or fortified yeast extract spread for vitamin B12.
3. Iodine-fortified foods or nori seaweed.
4. Rapeseed oil for cooking, walnuts, hemp drink and hemp seeds to provide ALA omega-3 fatty acids.
5. Fortified breakfast cereals for iron and B vitamins.
6. Nuts, nut butters and seeds for a range of essential micronutrients.

Remember that you don't have to get all of it right from day one. You could decide to take an iodine supplement for now, with the goal to introduce more iodine-rich foods as you get used to your vegan savvy diet.

If you would rather take a supplement to safeguard you against nutritional deficiencies, these are the main supplements you need to consider daily[136]:

1. Vitamin D (10mcg), especially in autumn and winter
2. Vitamin B12 (10mcg)
3. Iodine (140mcg)
4. Omega-3 (250mg vegan DHA and EPA)
5. Selenium (60mcg for women or 75mcg for men)

This doesn't mean you need to take five pills – it might be easier to find one that gives you everything, just check the dosages aren't too high, especially for selenium and iodine.

Mind tiles

1.

Be gentle on yourself. There's lots to learn and it won't happen overnight.

2.

If you're eating better than you were yesterday, you're already winning.

3.

Every step you take brings you closer to the version of yourself you want to be.

4.

Notice, notice and notice! Simply observing your behaviour helps you change it.

5.

Surround yourself with people who are going to support you on this journey.

6.

Remember the power of a metaphor, like a song or picture that represents the new healthier you: they can transform your thinking instantly.

7.

Your emotions are your reality. Get in touch with your feelings; don't ignore them.

8.

Get smart! Use the tools and techniques in this book to propel you forwards.

9.

Pay attention to what your body is trying to tell you. It's got its own intelligence – listen to it.

All your nutrient bridges

The Nutrient Bridge is a realistic and practical tool to help you enrich your meals (see page 7). You don't need to be adding all bridges to your meals, just pick and choose which ones suit you for any given meal or snack. Each box is an example of how to create a savvy plate.

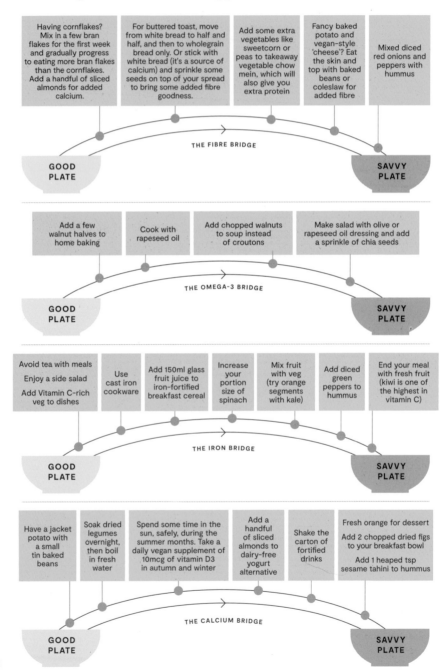

THE FIBRE BRIDGE

Having cornflakes? Mix in a few bran flakes for the first week and gradually progress to eating more bran flakes than the cornflakes. Add a handful of sliced almonds for added calcium.

For buttered toast, move from white bread to half and half, and then to wholegrain bread only. Or stick with white bread (it's a source of calcium) and sprinkle some seeds on top of your spread to bring some added fibre goodness.

Add some extra vegetables like sweetcorn or peas to takeaway vegetable chow mein, which will also give you extra protein

Fancy baked potato and vegan-style 'cheese'? Eat the skin and top with baked beans or coleslaw for added fibre

Mixed diced red onions and peppers with hummus

THE OMEGA-3 BRIDGE

Add a few walnut halves to home baking

Cook with rapeseed oil

Add chopped walnuts to soup instead of croutons

Make salad with olive or rapeseed oil dressing and add a sprinkle of chia seeds

THE IRON BRIDGE

Avoid tea with meals

Enjoy a side salad

Add Vitamin C-rich veg to dishes

Use cast iron cookware

Add 150ml glass fruit juice to iron-fortified breakfast cereal

Increase your portion size of spinach

Mix fruit with veg (try orange segments with kale)

Add diced green peppers to hummus

End your meal with fresh fruit (kiwi is one of the highest in vitamin C)

THE CALCIUM BRIDGE

Have a jacket potato with a small tin baked beans

Soak dried legumes overnight, then boil in fresh water

Spend some time in the sun, safely, during the summer months. Take a daily vegan supplement of 10mcg of vitamin D3 in autumn and winter

Add a handful of sliced almonds to dairy-free yogurt alternative

Shake the carton of fortified drinks

Fresh orange for dessert

Add 2 chopped dried figs to your breakfast bowl

Add 1 heaped tsp sesame tahini to hummus

GOOD PLATE

SAVVY PLATE

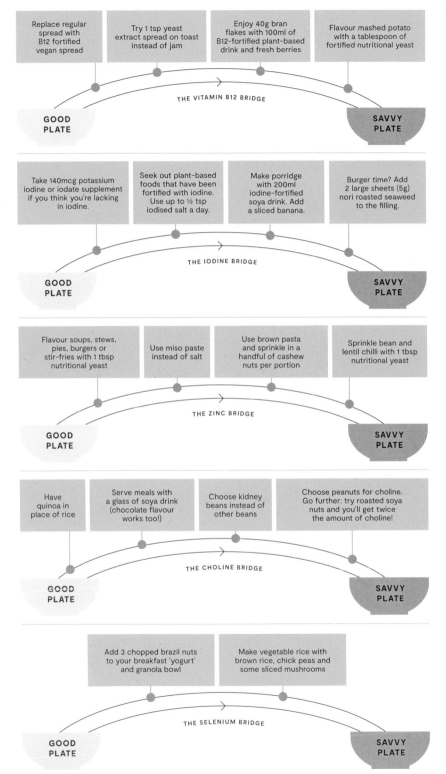

Replace regular spread with B12 fortified vegan spread

Try 1 tsp yeast extract spread on toast instead of jam

Enjoy 40g bran flakes with 100ml of B12-fortified plant-based drink and fresh berries

Flavour mashed potato with a tablespoon of fortified nutritional yeast

GOOD PLATE

SAVVY PLATE

THE VITAMIN B12 BRIDGE

Take 140mcg potassium iodine or iodate supplement if you think you're lacking in iodine.

Seek out plant-based foods that have been fortified with iodine. Use up to ½ tsp iodised salt a day.

Make porridge with 200ml iodine-fortified soya drink. Add a sliced banana.

Burger time? Add 2 large sheets (5g) nori roasted seaweed to the filling.

GOOD PLATE

SAVVY PLATE

THE IODINE BRIDGE

Flavour soups, stews, pies, burgers or stir-fries with 1 tbsp nutritional yeast

Use miso paste instead of salt

Use brown pasta and sprinkle in a handful of cashew nuts per portion

Sprinkle bean and lentil chilli with 1 tbsp nutritional yeast

GOOD PLATE

SAVVY PLATE

THE ZINC BRIDGE

Have quinoa in place of rice

Serve meals with a glass of soya drink (chocolate flavour works too!)

Choose kidney beans instead of other beans

Choose peanuts for choline. Go further: try roasted soya nuts and you'll get twice the amount of choline!

GOOD PLATE

SAVVY PLATE

THE CHOLINE BRIDGE

Add 3 chopped brazil nuts to your breakfast 'yogurt' and granola bowl

Make vegetable rice with brown rice, chick peas and some sliced mushrooms

GOOD PLATE

SAVVY PLATE

THE SELENIUM BRIDGE

FOOD	VVPC	PROTEIN	FIBRE	GOOD FATS	OMEGA-3 ALA	IRON
FRESH FRUIT AND VEGETABLES						
All fresh fruit and vegetables	V		✓			
Avocado	V		✓	✓		
Berries	V		✓			✓ [a]
Broccoli	V		✓			✓ [a]
Brussels sprouts	V		✓			✓ [a]
Carrots	V		✓			
Cauliflower	V		✓			
Beans, green	V		✓			
Fruit juice, citrus, unsweetened	V					✓ [a]
Green leafy vegetables	V		✓		✓	
Kale	V		✓			✓
Kiwi fruit	V		✓			✓ [a]
Mushrooms, white	V		✓			
Okra	V		✓			
Oranges	V		✓			✓ [a]
Pak choi	V		✓			
Peas, fresh	V	✓	✓			✓
Pears	V		✓			
Peppers	V		✓			✓ [a]
Potatoes (with skin)	V	✓	✓			
Shiitake mushrooms	V		✓			
Spinach	V		✓			✓
Spring greens	V		✓			✓
Sweetcorn	V	✓	✓			
Tomatoes	V		✓			
Watercress	V		✓			
VEGETABLES, FROZEN						
Beans, Edamame	V	✓	✓		✓	

VITAMIN B12	CALCIUM	OTHER B VITAMINS	IODINE	ZINC	CHOLINE	SELENIUM
		✓				
		✓				
	✓	✓			✓	
		✓			✓	
		✓			✓	
		✓				
	✓	✓				
	✓✓	✓				
				✓	✓	✓✓
	✓	✓				
	✓	✓			✓	
	✓	✓				
		✓			✓	
		✓			✓	
					✓	
		✓	✓			✓
	✓	✓				
		✓				
		✓				
	✓	✓				
		✓		✓	✓	

KEY

✓✓ indicates a significant source of micronutrients or omega-3 fatty acids
a helps absorption
b depends on brand

c Although sunflower seeds contain good fats, they are rich in omega-6 fatty acids, which could hamper your body's levels of omega-3 fatty acids, so you won't see a tick for good fats on this table.

FOOD	VVPC	PROTEIN	FIBRE	GOOD FATS	OMEGA-3 ALA	IRON
Green leafy vegetables	V		✓		✓	
Peas	V	✓	✓			✓
Spinach	V		✓			✓✓
Sweetcorn	V	✓	✓			
DRIED FRUIT						
Apricots	V		✓			✓
Figs	V		✓			✓
Prunes	V		✓			✓
Raisins	V		✓			✓
BEANS AND PULSES, DRIED						
Beans, all	P	✓	✓			✓
Chickpeas	P	✓	✓			✓
Lentils	P	✓	✓			✓
Beans, red kidney	P	✓	✓			✓
BEANS AND PULSES, CANNED						
Beans, all	P	✓	✓			✓
Baked beans in tomato sauce	P	✓	✓			✓✓
Chickpeas	P	✓	✓			✓
Lentils	P	✓	✓			✓
Lentil soup	V		✓			✓
Beans, red kidney	P	✓	✓			✓
Sweetcorn, canned	V	✓	✓			
CHILLED FOODS						
Meat substitutes						
Mycoprotein (sold as Quorn™) and products made from this	P	✓	✓			
Seitan (wheat gluten) meat substitute and products made from this	P	✓	✓			
Soya-based meat substitutes	P	✓	✓			
Tempeh	P	✓	✓			✓✓
Tofu	P	✓				✓
Products made from tofu	P	✓				
Dairy alternatives (fortification varies by brand)						
Non-dairy spreads fortified with omega-3 fatty acids and B vitamins					✓	

VITAMIN B12	CALCIUM	OTHER B VITAMINS	IODINE	ZINC	CHOLINE	SELENIUM
	✓	✓				
		✓			✓	
		✓	✓			
		✓				
	✓					
		✓		✓		✓✓
		✓		✓		✓
		✓		✓	✓	
	✓			✓		✓
		✓		✓		✓✓
		✓		✓		✓
		✓		✓	✓	
		✓				
	✓✓			✓✓		
	✓✓			✓	✓	✓
	✓					
✓		✓				

FOOD	VVPC	PROTEIN	FIBRE	GOOD FATS	OMEGA-3 ALA	IRON
Plant-based cheese alternative, fortified						
Plant-based drink, chocolate, fortified						
Plant-based drink, oat, fortified						
Plant-based drink, soya, fortified	P	✓				
Plant-based drink, hemp, not fortified					✓	
Plant-based drink, soya, not fortified	P	✓				
Plant-based drinks, other (e.g. almond, coconut, hazelnut, rice), fortified						
Plant-based yogurt alternative, coconut, fortified						
Plant-based yogurt alternative, soya, fortified	P	✓				
Dips						
Hummus	P	✓	✓			✓
NUTS						
Almonds	P	✓	✓	✓		✓
Brazil nuts	P	✓	✓	✓		✓
Cashew nuts	P	✓	✓	✓		✓
Hazelnuts	P	✓	✓	✓		✓
Peanuts	P	✓	✓	✓		✓
Walnuts	P	✓	✓	✓	✓✓	✓
SEEDS						
Chia seeds	P	✓	✓	✓	✓✓	✓
Flax seeds (linseeds)	P	✓	✓	✓	✓✓	✓
Hemp seeds	P	✓	✓	✓	✓✓	✓
Pumpkin seeds	P	✓	✓			✓✓
Sesame seeds	P	✓	✓	✓		✓✓
Sunflower seeds[c]	P	✓	✓			✓
NUT AND SEED BUTTERS						
Almond butter	P	✓	✓	✓		✓
Peanut butter	P	✓	✓	✓		✓
Sesame tahini	P	✓	✓	✓		✓
BREAD						
Pitta, wholemeal	C	✓	✓			

VITAMIN B12	CALCIUM	OTHER B VITAMINS	IODINE	ZINC	CHOLINE	SELENIUM
✓✓b						
✓b	✓✓				✓	
✓✓	✓✓	✓	✓✓b			
✓✓	✓✓	✓	✓✓b		✓	✓
					✓	✓
✓✓	✓✓	✓				
✓b	✓✓b					
✓✓b	✓✓					
		✓		✓		
	✓				✓	
				✓		✓✓
		✓		✓✓		✓✓
		✓				
		✓		✓	✓	
		✓		✓		
	✓	✓		✓		✓
		✓		✓		
		✓		✓		
		✓		✓✓	✓	
	✓✓	✓		✓		
	✓	✓		✓✓	✓	✓✓
	✓				✓	
		✓		✓	✓	
	✓✓	✓				

FOOD	VVPC	PROTEIN	FIBRE	GOOD FATS	OMEGA-3 ALA	IRON
Soya and linseed	C	✓	✓		✓✓	
White	C	✓				✓
Wholemeal	C	✓	✓			✓✓

BREAKFAST CEREALS (FORTIFICATION VARIES BY BRAND)

FOOD	VVPC	PROTEIN	FIBRE	GOOD FATS	OMEGA-3 ALA	IRON
All fortified breakfast cereals	C					✓✓
Bran flakes, fortified	C		✓			✓✓
Instant oat cereal, fortified	C		✓			✓✓
Malted flake cereal, fortified	C		✓			✓✓
Malted wheat cereal, fortified	C		✓			✓✓
Muesli	C		✓			✓
Porridge oats	C	✓	✓			✓
Wheat biscuits breakfast cereal, fortified	C		✓			✓✓

GRAINS (E.G. RICE AND PASTA)

FOOD	VVPC	PROTEIN	FIBRE	GOOD FATS	OMEGA-3 ALA	IRON
Couscous	C	✓				✓
Quinoa	C	✓	✓			✓✓
Rice, brown	C	✓	✓			✓
Pasta, white	C	✓				✓
Pasta, wholewheat	C	✓	✓			✓✓

NUTRITIOUS FLAVOURINGS

FOOD	VVPC	PROTEIN	FIBRE	GOOD FATS	OMEGA-3 ALA	IRON
Iodised salt (as part of daily 6g salt limit)						
Lemon juice						✓ [a]
Miso						✓
Nori seaweed (sushi sheets)						✓
Nutritional yeast flakes, fortified		✓				
Yeast extract, fortified						

OILS

FOOD	VVPC	PROTEIN	FIBRE	GOOD FATS	OMEGA-3 ALA	IRON
Olive				✓		
Rapeseed				✓	✓✓	

OTHER

FOOD	VVPC	PROTEIN	FIBRE	GOOD FATS	OMEGA-3 ALA	IRON
Chocolate, dark (70% cocoa solids)						✓
Oatcakes	C	✓	✓			✓
Sesame snaps		✓	✓			
Twiglets (savoury whole wheat sticks)	C		✓			

BEYOND
THE BOOK

VITAMIN B12	CALCIUM	OTHER B VITAMINS	IODINE	ZINC	CHOLINE	SELENIUM
	✓✓					
	✓✓	✓				✓
	✓	✓		✓		✓
		✓				
✓✓		✓				
✓✓	✓✓	✓				
✓✓		✓				
✓✓		✓				
		✓				
		✓		✓		
		✓				
				✓		✓
		✓		✓✓	✓	✓
		✓		✓✓		✓✓
				✓		✓✓
				✓✓		✓✓
			✓✓			
				✓		
✓✓			✓✓			
✓✓		✓		✓✓		
✓✓		✓				
	✓					
		✓				

Putting it all together, one step at a time

Choose one thing that you want to focus on. It's virtually impossible to take on a healthier eating plan by doing everything from the word go. It's not necessary either. Here are some tips to help you decide which areas to focus on:

1. If you've recently become vegan and are looking for nutritious dairy alternatives, go back to the tips in chapter 8 on calcium and make this your first goal.
2. If you're constantly feeling hungry, make sure you've covered your protein and fibre needs (chapters 4 and 5) before moving on to other nutrients.
3. If you're struggling with your weight, you might prefer to focus on picturing your VVPC plate (chapter 2) to help keep an eye on your portion sizes.
4. Feeling tired? You may decide that all you want to do for a couple of weeks is to look for iron and B vitamin fixes (see chapter 7).
5. If you're bored of eating the same vegetables, brighten up your meals with more colour – the tips in chapter 3 are made especially for you.
6. If it's party season, jump to the Eating Out chapter.
7. Beans and lentils not your thing? Check out other nutritious ways to get your protein (see page 40).
8. Love cooking but not sure how healthy your recipes are? Look at the ingredients and see how they match up to the recommended ones in the Master Shopping and Nutrient Guide (see pages 160–167). Maybe you could create your own Nutrient Bridges for your favourite recipes?

You'll find lots of vegan sav vy resources and blogs
on www.azminanutrition.com

Lastly, tell me how you're doing! Write to me via azminanutrition.com or on @AzminaNutrition on Twitter and Instagram.

'Transformation can happen in an instant. Sometimes it takes a little longer.'

I have no conflicts of interest in writing this book. You'll see that I may refer to a food brand on occasion to illustrate how you can get certain nutrients. I do not favour any of these brands apart from the fact that they may offer you nutritional benefits. I have not been compensated (financially or otherwise) or influenced by any brands or commercial organisations at the time of writing this book.

The food and nutrient content charts in this book are intended to help you make informed food choices. The charts or shopping lists do not necessarily represent what's called a 'significant amount' of a given nutrient. 'Significant amount' for vitamins and minerals means 15% of that nutrient's RI per 100g (or single serving) of food.

The shopping lists in this book are meant as a general guide only. Some foods are concentrated sources of nutrients but are usually consumed in small quantities (e.g. seeds). Conversely, other foods contain lower concentrations of nutrients but can still make a useful contribution to overall nutrient intake owing to the larger quantities consumed (e.g. pasta) or because they are often consumed alongside other foods that are also useful sources (e.g. baked beans on toast). Therefore, a wide range of foods are included in the tables and shopping lists to provide information that is as helpful as possible.

All the nutrition composition figures are correct at the time of writing. Most analysis is based on widely accepted professional data sources, as referenced. A few are indicated as manufacturers' product data; these may change if product formulations change, so if you read the book at a later date, check labels for a more accurate picture.

The dietary advice in this book is aimed at the general public and is not intended to be a substitute for personalised dietary advice by a registered dietitian or registered nutritionist. Look for the letters RD or RNutr respectively after an experts name to give you that extra peace of mind that they are properly qualified.

FOR HEALTHCARE PROFESSIONALS

Images and diagrams are intended to illustrate scientific concepts in a simple way and are not meant to convey the entirety of any of the principles behind the evidence.

When used in relation to nutrition claims in commercial settings, the term 'source' is associated with specific criteria (e.g. providing at least 15% of the Reference Intake of a vitamin or mineral). However, throughout this book, I have used the term 'source' in a more generic sense in line with its dictionary definition ('a place, person, or thing from which something originates or can be obtained'). Its use is not intended to imply that a food contains sufficient levels of a nutrient to meet the criteria for a 'source of' nutrition claim.

In the tables and shopping list, the term 'significant sources' has been used to indicate foods for which the specified serving would provide at least 15% of the Reference Intake for that nutrient. The term 'other useful sources' has been used to indicate foods that are generally accepted sources of a nutrient and/or that can help an individual to achieve recommended intakes, particularly for nutrients that tend to be less abundant in plant-based foods.

Generally accepted sources include foods highlighted in reliable reference sources including (but not limited to) NHS Digital and The Vegan Society.

Sources of key nutrients are highlighted throughout the book, but this is not intended to be a comprehensive listing. Other foods may also provide useful amounts of these nutrients. Reference information on the levels of these nutrients in commonly consumed foods can be accessed at: https://quadram.ac.uk/UKfoodcomposition/ .

Where possible, nutrient values are taken from the UK reference dataset, McCance & Widdowson's The Composition of Foods, accessed via The Composition of Foods Integrated Dataset (https://www.gov.uk/government/publications/composition-of-foods-integrated-dataset-cofid). Where necessary, other data sources were used, in particular, manufacturers' data and the US reference dataset, accessed via FoodData Central (https://fdc.nal.usda.gov/index.html).

References

1 Nudge-it (Accessed May 2020). Nudging Consumers toward Healthier Choices. https://www.nudge-it.eu/topics/nudging-the-consumer-toward-healthier-choices.html

2 Zellner DA, Siemers E, Teran V, et al (2011) 'Neatness counts. How plating affects liking for the taste of food'. Appetite, 57: 642-648. 10.1016/j.appet.2011.08.004'

3 Nudge-it (Accessed May 2020). 'Nudging Consumers toward Healthier Choices. https://www.nudge-it.eu/topics/nudging-the-consumer-toward-healthier-choices.html

4 Glycemic Index Foundation (2017, Accessed May 2020). 'Top Tips to go Low GI'. https://www.gisymbol.com/top-tips-to-go-low-gi/

5 OHSU Knight Cardiovascular Institute (Accessed May 2020). 'My Heart Healthy Plate'. Oregon Health & Science University. https://www.ohsu.edu/knight-cardiovascular-institute/my-heart-healthy-plate

6 Umass Medical School (2018). 'Healthy Eating is Important for Diabetes Management and Glucose Control'. https://www.umassmed.edu/dcoe/diabetes-education/nutrition/

7 Government of Canada (2020). Canada's Food Guide. https://food-guide.canada.ca/en/

8 The Vegetarian Resource Group (Accessed May 2020). 'My Vegan Plate'. https://www.vrg.org/nutshell/MyVeganPlate.pdf

9 Govindji A and Puddefoot N (2004). 'The GI Plan: Lose weight forever'. Vermilion.

10 Umass Medical School (Accessed May 2020). 'The Zimbabwe Hand Jive: A Simple Method of Portion Portion Control'. https://www.umassmed.edu/dcoe/diabetes-education/nutrition/zimbabwe-hand-jive/

11 Aune D, Giovannucci E, Boffetta P, et al (2017). 'Fruit and vegetable intake and the risk of cardiovascular disease, total cancer and all-cause mortality—a systematic review and dose-response meta-analysis of prospective studies'. International Journal of Epidemiology. Volume 46, Issue 3, June 2017, Pages 1029–1056 https://doi.org/10.1093/ije/dyw319

12 European Commission (Accessed May 2020). EU Register of nutrition and health claims made on food. https://ec.europa.eu/food/safety/labelling_nutrition/claims/register/public/?event=register.home

13 The Vegan RD (Accessed May 2020). 'Plant Protein: A Vegan Nutrition Primer'. https://www.theveganrd.com/vegan-nutrition-101/vegan-nutrition-primers/plant-protein-a-vegan-nutrition-primer/

14 Vegetarian Nutrition (2019). 'Protein in Vegetarian and Vegan Diets'. https://vegetariannutrition.net/docs/Protein-Vegetarian-Nutrition.pdf

15 Finnigan, T., Wall, B. T., Wilde, P. J., et al. (2019). 'Mycoprotein: The Future of Nutritious Nonmeat Protein, a Symposium Review'. Current developments in nutrition, 3(6), nzz021. https://doi.org/10.1093/cdn/nzz021

16 The Vegetarian Society (Accessed May 2020). 'Protein: what food is protein in?'. https://www.vegsoc.org/info-hub/health-and-nutrition/protein/

17 Vegan Health (February 2020). 'Protein Part 2: Research'. https://veganhealth.org/protein-part-2/#protein-foods

18 McCance & Widdowson (2019). 'Composition of foods integrated dataset (CoFID). https://www.gov.uk/government/publications/composition-of-foods-integrated-dataset-cofid.

19 Rizzo G & Baroni L (2018). 'Soy, Soy Foods and Their Role in Vegetarian Diets'. Nutrients 10(1). pii: E43.

20 D'Adamo C.R and Sahin A (2014) 'Soy foods and supplementation: A review of commonly perceived health benefits and risks'. Altern. Ther. Health Med. 2014; 20:39–51

21 Vegan Health (February 2020). 'Protein Part 2: Research'. https://veganhealth.org/protein-part-1/#recommendations

22 European Commission (Accessed May 2020). EU Register of nutrition and health claims made on food. https://ec.europa.eu/food/safety/labelling_nutrition/claims/register/public/?event=register.home

23 British Nutrition Foundation (2018). 'Dietary Fibre'. https://www.nutrition.org.uk/nutritionscience/nutrients-food-and-ingredients/dietary-fibre.html?start=1

24 Scientific Advisory Committee on Nutrition (2015).

'Carbohydrates and Health'. https://assets.publishing.service.gov.uk/government/uploads/system/uploads/attachment_data/file/445503/SACN_Carbohydrates_and_Health.pdf

25 BDA The Association of UK Dietitians (2019). 'What is Fibre?' https://www.bda.uk.com/resource/fibre.html

26 British Nutrition Foundation (2018). 'Dietary Fibre'. https://www.nutrition.org.uk/nutritionscience/nutrients-food-and-ingredients/dietary-fibre.html?start=3

27 Scientific Advisory Committee on Nutrition (2019). 'Saturated Fats and Health'. https://assets.publishing.service.gov.uk/government/uploads/system/uploads/attachment_data/file/814995/SACN_report_on_saturated_fat_and_health.pdf

28 Benatar, J. R., & Stewart, R. (2018). 'Cardiometabolic risk factors in vegans; A meta-analysis of observational studies'. PloS one, 13(12), e0209086. https://doi.org/10.1371/journal.pone.0209086

29 European Commission (Accessed May 2020). EU Register of nutrition and health claims made on food. https://ec.europa.eu/food/safety/labelling_nutrition/claims/register/

30 Saunders AV, Davis BC, Garg ML (2013) 'Omega-3 polyunsaturated fatty acids and vegetarian diets'. Med J Aust 199(S4):S22-6.

31 Shahidi F, Ambigaipalan P. 'Omega-3 Polyunsaturated Fatty Acids and Their Health Benefits'. Annu Rev Food Sci Technol. 2018;9:345-381. doi:10.1146/annurev-food-111317-095850

32 Bradbury J. 'Docosahexaenoic acid (DHA): an ancient nutrient for the modern human brain'. Nutrients. 2011;3(5):529-554. doi:10.3390/nu3050529

33 The Vegan Society (Accessed May 2020). 'Omega-3 and omega-6 fats'. https://www.vegansociety.com/resources/nutrition-and-health/nutrients/omega-3-and-omega-6-fats

34 European Food Safety Authority (2019). DRV Finder. https://www.efsa.europa.eu/en/interactive-pages/drvs

35 European Food Safety Authority (2017). 'Overview on Dietary Reference Values for the EU population as derived by the EFSA Panel on Dietetic Products, Nutrition and Allergies (NDA)'. https://www.efsa.europa.eu/sites/default/files/assets/DRV_Summary_tables_jan_17.pdf

36 National Institutes of Health (2019). 'Omega-3 Fatty Acids'. https://ods.od.nih.gov/factsheets/Omega3FattyAcids-HealthProfessional/

37 Burns-Whitmore B, Froyen E, Heskey C, et al (2019) 'Alpha-Linolenic and Linoleic Fatty Acids in the Vegan Diet: Do They Require Dietary Reference Intake/Adequate Intake Special Consideration?'. Nutrients. 2019;11(10):2365. Published 2019 Oct 4. doi:10.3390/nu11102365

38 The Scientific Advisory Committee (2019). 'Saturated Fats and Health'. https://www.gov.uk/government/publications/saturated-fats-and-health-sacn-report

39 Ginsberg, H. N., Karmally, W., Siddiqui, M., et al. (1995). 'Increases in dietary cholesterol are associated with modest increases in both LDL and HDL cholesterol in healthy young women'. Arteriosclerosis, thrombosis, and vascular biology, 15(2), 169–178. https://doi.org/10.1161/01.atv.15.2.169

40 Ginsberg, H. N., Karmally, W., Siddiqui, M., et al. (1994). 'A dose-response study of the effects of dietary cholesterol on fasting and postprandial lipid and lipoprotein metabolism in healthy young men'. Arteriosclerosis and thrombosis : a journal of vascular biology, 14(4), 576–586. https://doi.org/10.1161/01.atv.14.4.576

41 McCance & Widdowson (2019). 'Composition of foods integrated dataset (CoFID). https://www.gov.uk/government/publications/composition-of-foods-integrated-dataset-cofid

42 Taylor, V (Accessed May 2020). 'I've heard coconut oil is good for you. Is this true?' British Heart Foundation Heart Matters. https://www.bhf.org.uk/informationsupport/heart-matters-magazine/nutrition/ask-the-expert/coconut-oil

43 HEART UK (Accessed May 2020). 'HEART UK says BBC coconut oil claim not to be trusted.' https://www.heartuk.org.uk/news/latest/post/16-heart-uk-says-bbc-coconut-oil-claim-not-to-be-trusted

44 NHS (Accessed May 2020). 'Fat: the facts.' https://www.nhs.uk/live-well/eat-well/different-fats-nutrition/

45 Lockyer S and Stanner S (2016). 'Coconut oil: a nutty idea?' British Nutrition Foundation. Nutrition Bulletin 41, 42–54 https://onlinelibrary.wiley.com/doi/full/10.1111/nbu.12188

46 Ghavami A, Coward WA, Bluck LJ. The effect of food preparation on the bioavailability of carotenoids from carrots using intrinsic labelling. Br J Nutr. 2012;107(9):1350-1366. doi:10.1017/S000711451100451X

47 Davey GK, Spencer EA, Appleby PN, et al. EPIC-Oxford: lifestyle characteristics and nutrient intakes in a cohort of 33 883 meat-eaters and 31 546 non meat-eaters in the UK. Public Health Nutr. 2003;6(3):259-269. doi:10.1079/PHN2002430

48 European Commission (Accessed May 2020). EU Register of nutrition and health claims made on food. https://ec.europa.eu/food/safety/labelling_nutrition/claims/register/public/?event=register.home

49 BDA The Association of UK Dietitians (2017). 'Iron: Food Fact Sheet.'https://www.bda.uk.com/resource/iron-rich-foods-iron-deficiency.html

50 Public Health England (2018) National Diet and Nutrition Survey Results from Years 7 and 8 (combined) of the Rolling Programme (2014/2015 to 2015/2016) https://assets.publishing.service.gov.uk/government/uploads/system/uploads/attachment_data/file/699241/NDNS_results_years_7_and_8.pdf

51 McCance & Widdowson (2019). 'Composition of foods integrated dataset (CoFID). https://www.gov.uk/government/publications/composition-of-foods-integrated-dataset-cofid

52 University of Hawai'i at Mānoa Food Science and Human Nutrition Program, Open Library (2011). 'Human Nutrition: iron.' https://ecampusontario.pressbooks.pub/humannutrition/chapter/iron/

53 Hallberg L. Wheat fiber, phytates and iron absorption. Scand J Gastroenterol Suppl. 1987;129:73-79. doi:10.3109/00365528709095855

54 Hallberg L, Brune M, Rossander L. 'The role of vitamin C in iron absorption'. Int J Vitam Nutr Res Suppl. 1989;30:103-108. https://www.ncbi.nlm.nih.gov/pubmed/2507689

55,56 Ole Haagen Nielsen, Christoffer Soendergaard, Malene Elbaek Vikner, Gunter Weiss (2018). 'Rational Management of Iron-Deficiency Anaemia in Inflammatory Bowel Disease.'56. Nielson OH et al (2018). 'Rational Management of Iron-Deficiency Anaemia in Inflammatory Bowel Disease'. https://www.mdpi.com/2072-6643/10/1/82/htm

57 Iron Disorders Institute (Updated 2020). 'Achieving Iron Balance with Diet. http://www.irondisorders.org/diet/

58 Scrimshaw NS. Iron deficiency [published correction appears in Sci Am 1992 Jan;266(1):following 8]. Sci Am. 1991;265(4):46-52. doi:10.1038/scientificamerican1091-46

59 Delimont, N. M., Haub, M. D., & Lindshield, B. L. (2017). 'The Impact of Tannin Consumption on Iron Bioavailability and Status: A Narrative Review'. Current developments in nutrition, 1(2), 1-12. https://doi.org/10.3945/cdn.116.000042/

60 Scientific Advisory Committee on Nutrition (2010). 'Iron and Health.' https://assets.publishing.service.gov.uk/government/uploads/system/uploads/attachment_data/file/339309/SACN_Iron_and_Health_Report.pdf

61 Geerligs PD, Brabin BJ, Omari AA (2003). Food prepared in iron cooking pots as an intervention for reducing iron deficiency anaemia in developing countries: a systematic review. J Hum Nutr Diet;16(4):275-281. doi:10.1046/j.1365-277x.2003.00447.x

62 Alves C, Saleh A, Alaofe H (2019). 'Iron-containing cookware for the reduction of iron deficiency anemia among children and females of reproductive age in low- and middle-income countries: A systematic review.' https://journals.plos.org/plosone/article?id=10.1371/journal.pone.0221094

63 Public Health England (2018). 'Campaign launches to help adults tackle "calorie creep."' https://phe-newsroom.prgloo.com/news/embargoed-phe-press-release-400-600-600-campaign-launches-to-help-adults-tackle-calorie-creep

64, 65 Public Health England (2016). 'Government recommendations for energy and nutrients for males and females aged 1-18 years and 19+ years.' https://assets.publishing.service.gov.uk/government/uploads/system/uploads/attachment_data/file/618167/government_dietary_recommendations.pdf

66 Spencer EA, Appleby PN, Davey GK, et al (2003). Diet and body mass index in 38000 EPIC-Oxford meat-eaters, fish-eaters, vegetarians and vegans. Int J Obes Relat Metab Disord;27(6):728-734. doi:10.1038/sj.ijo.0802300

67 Vegan Society (2020). 'Vegan Eatwell Guide.' https://www.vegansociety.com/sites/default/files/uploads/downloads/The%20Vegan%20Eatwell%20Guide_1.pdf

68 Department of Health (1991). 'Dietary Reference Values for Food Energy and Nutrients for the United Kingdom.' HMSO

69 Public Health England (2019). 'National Diet and Nutrition Survey Years 1 to 9 of the Rolling Programme (2008/9-2016/17): Time trend and income analyses'. https://assets.publishing.service.gov.uk/government/uploads/system/uploads/attachment_data/file/772434/NDNS_UK_Y1-9_report.pdf

70 British Nutrition Foundation (2018). 'Summary of Key Findings from the NDNS Report of Years 7 and 8.' https://www.nutrition.org.uk/nutritioninthenews/new-reports/ndnsyears7and8.html

71 New SA (2003/4). Intake of fruit and vegetables: implications for bone health [published correction appears in Proc Nutr Soc. 2004 Feb;63(1):187]. Proc Nutr Soc. 2003;62(4):889-899. doi:10.1079/PNS2003310

72 Średnicka-Tober D, Barański M, Seal CJ, et al (2016). Higher PUFA and n-3 PUFA, conjugated linoleic acid, ●-tocopherol and iron, but lower iodine and selenium concentrations in organic milk: a systematic literature review and meta- and redundancy analyses. Br J Nutr;115(6):1043-1060. doi:10.1017/S0007114516000349

73 Official Journal of the European Union (2013). REGULATION (EU) No 1308/2013 OF THE EUROPEAN PARLIAMENT AND OF THE COUNCIL of 17 December 2013 establishing a common organisation of the markets in agricultural products and repealing Council Regulations (EEC) No 922/72, (EEC) No 234/79, (EC) No 1037/2001 and (EC) No 1234/2007. https://eur-lex.europa.eu/LexUriServ/LexUriServ.do?uri=OJ:L:2013:347:0671:0854:EN:PDF

74 Heaney RP, Dowell MS, Rafferty K et al (2000). Bioavailability of the calcium in fortified soy imitation milk, with some observations on method. Am J Clin Nutrition.;71(5):1166-1169. doi:10.1093/ajcn/71.5.1166

75 Zhao Y, Martin BR, Weaver CM. Calcium bioavailability of calcium carbonate fortified soymilk is equivalent to cow's milk in young women. J Nutr. 2005;135(10):2379-2382. doi:10.1093/jn/135.10.2379

76 Heaney RP, Rafferty K (2006). 'The settling problem in calcium-fortified soybean drinks'. J Am Diet Assoc.;106(11):1753-1755. doi:10.1016/j.jada.2006.08.008

77 McCance & Widdowson (2019). 'Composition of foods integrated dataset (CoFID). https://www.gov.uk/government/publications/composition-of-foods-integrated-dataset-cofid

78 U.S. Department of Agriculture, Agricultural Research Service. FoodData Central, 2019. fdc.nal.usda.gov

79 Heaney RP, Dowell MS, Rafferty K, Bierman J (2000). 'Bioavailability of the calcium in fortified soy imitation milk, with some observations on method'. Am J Clin Nutr.;71(5):1166-1169. doi:10.1093/ajcn/71.5.1166

80 Nielson OH Soendergaard C, Vikner ME et al (2018). 'Rational Management of Iron-Deficiency Anaemia in Inflammatory Bowel Disease'. Nutrients, 10(1), 82; https://doi.org/10.3390/nu10010082

81 Noonan SC, Savage GP. Oxalate content of foods and its effect on humans. Asia Pac J Clin Nutr. 1999;8(1):64-74.

82 BDA The Association of UK Dietitians (2018). One Blue Dot 'Eating patterns for health and environmental sustainability: A Reference Guide for Dietitians'. https://www.bda.uk.com/uploads/assets/539e2268-7991-4d24-b9ee867c1b2808fc/421de049-2c41-4d85-934f0a2f6362cc4a/one%20blue%20dot%20reference%20guide.pdf

83 Dairy Nutrition (2020). 'Calcium and Bioavailability.' https://www.dairynutrition.ca/nutrients-in-milk-products/calcium/calcium-and-bioavailability

84 Gibson R. (1994). 'Content and bioavailability of trace elements in vegetarian diets.' Am J Clin Nutr.;59(5 Suppl):1223S-32S.

85 Kumar, A., & Kaur, S. (2017). Calcium: A Nutrient in Pregnancy. Journal of obstetrics and gynaecology of India, 67(5), 313-318. https://doi.org/10.1007/s13224-017-1007-2

86 Cancer Research UK (2019). 'Sun and Vitamin D.' https://

www.cancerresearchuk.org/about-cancer/causes-of-cancer/sun-uv-and-cancer/sun-and-vitamin-d

87　Public Health England (2019). 'National Diet and Nutrition Survey Years 1 to 9 of the Rolling Programme (2008/9–2016/17): Time trend and income analyses'. https://assets.publishing.service.gov.uk/government/uploads/system/uploads/attachment_data/file/772434/NDNS_UK_Y1-9_report.pdf

88　Royal Osteoporosis Society (2019). https://theros.org.uk/information-and-support/looking-after-your-bones/nutrition-for-bones/are-there-any-foods-i-should-avoid

89　Gille D & Schmid A (2015). 'Vitamin B12 in meat and dairy products'.Nutr Rev 73(2):106-15.

91　Selinger E, Kühn T, Procházková M, Anděl M et al. Vitamin B12 Deficiency Is Prevalent Among Czech Vegans Who Do Not Use Vitamin B12 Supplements. Nutrients. 2019;11(12):3019. Published 2019 Dec 10. doi:10.3390/nu11123019

92　Public Health England (2016). 'Government recommendations for energy and nutrients for males and females aged 1-18 years and 19+ years.' https://assets.publishing.service.gov.uk/government/uploads/system/uploads/attachment_data/file/618167/government_dietary_recommendations.pdf

93　European Commission (2020). EU Register of nutrition and health claims made on food. https://ec.europa.eu/food/safety/labelling_nutrition/claims/register/public/?event=search

94　McCance & Widdowson (2019). 'Composition of foods integrated dataset (CoFID)'. https://www.gov.uk/government/publications/composition-of-foods-integrated-dataset-cofid

95　The Vegan Society (Accessed May 2020). 'Vitamin B12.' https://www.vegansociety.com/resources/nutrition-and-health/nutrients/vitamin-b12

96　The Vegan Society (2020). 'What Every Vegan Should Know about Vitamin B12.' https://www.vegansociety.com/resources/nutrition-and-health/nutrients/vitamin-b12/what-every-vegan-should-know-about-vitamin-b12

97　WHO, UNICEF, & ICCIDD (2007). 'Assessment of iodine deficiency disorders and monitoring their elimination based on a 2011 national study of 14-15year old girls.'

98　Bates, B., Lennox, A., Prentice, A., et al (2014). 'National Diet and Nutrition Survey, Results from Years 1-4 of the Rolling Programme.'

99　Ma W, He X, Braverman L. 'Iodine Content in Milk Alternatives'. Thyroid. 2016;26(9):1308-1310. doi:10.1089/thy.2016.0239

100　Brantsæter AL, Knutsen HK, Johansen NC, et al. 'Inadequate Iodine Intake in Population Groups Defined by Age, Life Stage and Vegetarian Dietary Practice in a Norwegian Convenience Sample'. Nutrients. 2018;10(2):230. Published 2018 Feb 17. doi:10.3390/nu10020230

101　Leung AM, Lamar A, He X, Braverman LE, et al (2011). 'Iodine status and thyroid function of Boston-area vegetarians and vegans'. J Clin Endocrinol Metab. 96(8):E1303-E1307. doi:10.1210/jc.2011-0256

102　EFSA (2014). 'Scientific Opinion on Dietary Reference Values for iodine EFSA Panel on Dietetic Products, Nutrition and Allergies'. (NDA)2,3 12(5):3660.

103　Hypothyroidism. Bethesda, MD (2012). 'National Endocrine and Metabolic Diseases Information Service, US Dept of Health and Human Services.' NIH Publication No. 12-6180

104　Bath SC, Steer CD, Golding J, et al (2013). 'Effect of inadequate iodine status in UK pregnant women on cognitive outcomes in their children: results from the Avon Longitudinal Study of Parents and Children.' Lancet; 382:331-337. [PubMed: 23706508

105　Public Health England (2016) 'Government recommendations for energy and nutrients for males and females aged 1 – 18 years and 19+ years'. PHE: London. https://assets.publishing.service.gov.uk/government/uploads/system/uploads/attachment_data/file/618167/government_dietary_recommendations.pdf

106　Public Health England (2015/16). 'Years 7 to 8 of the Rolling Programme: Time trend and income analyse's. https://assets.publishing.service.gov.uk/government/uploads/

system/uploads/attachment_data/file/699241/NDNS_results_years_7_and_8.pdf

107　McCance & Widdowson (2019). 'Composition of foods integrated dataset (CoFID)'. https://www.gov.uk/government/publications/composition-of-foods-integrated-dataset-cofid

108　Bath, S. C., Hill, S., Infante, H. G., et al. (2017). 'Iodine concentration of milk-alternative drinks available in the UK in comparison with cows' milk'. The British journal of nutrition, 118(7), 525–532. https://doi.org/10.1017/S0007114517002136

109　Action on Salt (2020). 'Salt and Your Health.' http://www.actiononsalt.org.uk/salthealth/

110　BDA The Association of UK Dietitians (2019). 'Iodine: Food Fact Sheet.' https://www.bda.uk.com/resource/iodine.html

111　The Vegan Society (2020). 'Vegan Eatwell Guide.' https://www.vegansociety.com/sites/default/files/uploads/downloads/The%20Vegan%20Eatwell%20Guide_2.pdf

112　European Commission (2020). EU Register of nutrition and health claims made on food.

113　Public Health England (2016). 'Government recommendations for energy and nutrients for males and females aged 1-18 years and 19+ years.' https://assets.publishing.service.gov.uk/government/uploads/system/uploads/attachment_data/file/618167/government_dietary_recommendations.pdf

114　Gibson RS, Heath AL, Szymlek-Gay EA (2014). 'Is iron and zinc nutrition a concern for vegetarian infants and young children in industrialized countries?'. Am J Clin Nutr.;100 Suppl 1:459S-68S. doi:10.3945/ajcn.113.071241

115　Sandström B. 'Bioavailability of zinc'. Eur J Clin Nutr. 1997;51 Suppl 1:S17-S19.

116　EFSA (2014). 'Scientific Opinion on Dietary Reference Values for zinc EFSA Panel on Dietetic Products, Nutrition and Allergies.' https://efsa.onlinelibrary.wiley.com/doi/10.2903/j.efsa.2014.3844

117　Hills J (2019). 'Why You Need to Soak Nuts and Seeds Overnight in Water Before Eating Them'. Healthy and Natural World. https://www.healthyandnaturalworld.com/why-you-need-to-soak-nuts-and-seeds/

118　RGupta, R. K., Gangoliya, S. S., & Singh, N. K. (2015). 'Reduction of phytic acid and enhancement of bioavailable micronutrients in food grains'. Journal of food science and technology, 52(2), 676–684. https://doi.org/10.1007/s13197-013-0978-y

119　McCance & Widdowson (2019). 'Composition of foods integrated dataset (CoFID)'. https://www.gov.uk/government/publications/composition-of-foods-integrated-dataset-cofid

120　EFSA (2011) Scientific Opinion on the substantiation of health claims related to choline EFSA Panel on Dietetic Products, Nutrition and Allergies (NDA). EFSA Journal 9(4).

121　Schwarzenberg SJ, Georgieff MK and COMMITTEE ON NUTRITION. 'Advocacy for Improving Nutrition in the First 1000 Days to Support Childhood Development and Adult Health' Pediatrics February 2018, 141 (2) e20173716; DOI: https://doi.org/10.1542/peds.2017-3716

122　Derbyshire EJ (2019) 'Could we be Overlooking a Potential Choline Crisis in the United Kingdom'. BMJ Nutrition, Prevention & Health 1-4.

123　EFSA (2016) Dietary Reference Values for choline. EFSA Journal 14:4484.

124　EFSA Journal 2016;14(8):4484

125　Kim, S., Fenech, M.F. & Kim, P (2018). 'Nutritionally recommended food for semi- to strict vegetarian diets based on large-scale nutrient composition data'. Sci Rep 8, 4344. https://doi.org/10.1038/s41598-018-22691-1

126　LLewis ED, Kosik SJ, Zhao YY, et al (2014). 'Total choline and choline-containing moieties of commercially available pulses'. Plant Foods for Human Nutrition (Dordrecht, Netherlands); 69(2):115-121. DOI: 10.1007/s11130-014-0412-2.

127　McCance & Widdowson (2019). 'Composition of foods integrated dataset (CoFID)'. https://www.gov.uk/government/publications/composition-of-foods-integrated-dataset-cofid.

128　European Commission (2020). EU Register of nutrition and health claims made on food.

128 European Commission (2020). EU Register of nutrition and health claims made on food.

129 Mehdi Y, Hornick JL, Istasse L, et al (2013). 'Selenium in the environment, metabolism and involvement in body functions'. Molecules.;18(3):3292-3311. Published 2013 Mar 13. doi:10.3390/molecules18033292

130 British Nutrition Foundation (Accessed May 2020). 'Minerals and trace elements.' https://www.nutrition.org.uk/nutritionscience/nutrients-food-and-ingredients/minerals-and-trace-elements.html?limit=1&start=13

131 Derbyshire E. (2018). 'Micronutrient Intakes of British Adults Across Mid-Life: A Secondary Analysis of the UK National Diet and Nutrition Survey'. Frontiers in nutrition, 5, 55. https://doi.org/10.3389/fnut.2018.00055

132 Public Health England (2016). 'Government recommendations for energy and nutrients for males and females aged 1-18 years and 19+ years.'

133 McCance & Widdowson (2019). 'Composition of foods integrated dataset (CoFID)'. https://www.gov.uk/government/publications/composition-of-foods-integrated-dataset-cofid

134 The Vegan Society (2020). 'Selenium.' https://www.vegansociety.com/sites/default/files/uploads/downloads/Selenium%20PDF.pdf

135 Schaafsma G (2000), 'The Protein Digestibility-Corrected Amino Acid Score', The Journal of Nutrition, Volume 130, Issue 7, Pages 1865S–1867S, https://doi.org/10.1093/jn/130.7.1865S

136 The Vegan Society (2020). The Vegan Eatwell Guide. https://www.vegansociety.com/sites/default/files/uploads/downloads/The%20Vegan%20Eatwell%20Guide_2.pdf

Index

Acknowledgements

This book would not have been written if it wasn't for my daughter Shazia. She has been an inspiration and a role model. Shazia's big announcement that she had become vegan propelled me to learn and research so I could guide her better as a dietitian and a mother. So, I sought the advice of my trusted friend and dietitian, Smita Ganatra. We brainstormed how to create a simple model that was based on scientific principles but that could be communicated in a visual format. Thank you Smita for always being there for me.

I sought out Editorial Consultant Julia Kellaway, who polished my book proposal, so it met her high standards – and, as always, she was a joy to work with. My literary agent Jane Graham Maw 'got' me. She understood my need to get the facts right, to steer readers towards a realistic plan based on evidence, insight and simplicity. Sophie Allen, Commissioning Editor at Pavilion Books, came up with the winning formula – an illustrated book that conveyed nutrition in an accessible format. Sophie has been incredibly tolerant, taking on my challenges and requests for yet another design idea, yet another book title. Thank you, Sophie, for your patience and acceptance. And thank you to the design team at Evi O Studio for your creativity.

But the writing didn't just happen – I enlisted several experts to sense-check my translation of the science. A big thank you to esteemed dietitian Dr Frankie Phillips, Media Spokesperson for the British Dietetic Association, for her thorough peer-review and critique on significant aspects of the manuscript. Dr Emma Derbyshire, registered nutritionist and health writer, contributed her strong research skills regarding potential nutritional inadequacies in vegan diets. The work of expert dietitians who specialise in plant-based eating has helped me in my background research and I'd like to single two of them out here: Heather Russell and Jack Norris. There is extensive nutritional data in this book and my sincere gratitude goes to food composition expert and registered nutritionist Susan Church. Susan's high standards and diligence gave me peace of mind like no other.

Huge appreciation to Simone Schultz, for her keen eye and attention to detail. Not only did she provide professional editing skills and creativity, Simone was also one of my target audience 'check-points'. Thanks also to the twenty or so young professionals who shared their thinking on book titles, objectives and chapter headings; your views have helped provide a framework for my study.

And then – the biggest support of all – my family. Bizhan, your creative insights and breadth of thinking stretched my mind and gave me confidence. Our constant debating and discussions helped with design ideas and bringing the science to life. Shazia, you meticulously read every page to inform my writing and highlighted the issues you personally face on a vegan diet, helping me streamline my advice. I hope I have now equipped you better for your future food choices.

Devoting energy to this project has come at the expense of being less of a mother and wife over several long months. My husband Shamil, as with every significant project, has been my rock, the backbone that makes everything else fall into place. Not only has he relieved me of day-to-day domesticity, but his inquiring mind has challenged my writing exactly when I needed it. Thank you for your encouragement, patience and support, always.

A final thank you must go to Riel Sibley, whose idea it was to put my new-found knowledge into a book in the first place. If you hadn't planted that seed, this book may have been nothing more than a collection of yellow stickies by the side of my bed.

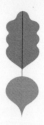

First published in the
United Kingdom in 2020 by Pavilion
43 Great Ormond Street
London
WC1N 3HZ

ISBN 978-1-91166-341-6
A CIP catalogue record for this book is available from the British Library.
10 9 8 7 6 5 4 3 2 1

Reproduction by Rival Colour, UK
Printed and bound by 1010 Printing International Ltd, China
www.pavilionbooks.com

Publisher: Helen Lewis
Commissioning editor: Sophie Allen
Design: Evi-O.Studio | Susan Le
Production manager: Phil Brown

MIX
Paper from
responsible sources
FSC® C016973

DISCLAIMERS: The information in this book is provided as an
information resource only and is not to be used or relied on for any
diagnostic, treatment or medical purpose. All health issues should be
discussed with your GP and/or other qualified medical professional.

Although the author and publisher have made every effort to ensure
that the information in this book is correct at press time, neither the
author nor the publisher takes responsibility or liability for any loss,
damage, claim or disruption caused by errors or omissions caused by
any reason, nor for any claim resulting from the use or misuse of the
information provided.

The following trademarks are mentioned in *Vegan Savvy* but the book
is not endorsed by any of the Trademark owners: Quorn, Engevita,
Marmite, Twiglets, Vegemite.

Epigraph credit (p4): Andre Agassi, OPEN (Harper Collins, 2010)